AF483526

Pharmaceutical Microbiology

A Laboratory Manual

Pharmaceutical Microbiology

A Laboratory Manual

Dr. G. Shyam Prasad

Assistant Professor
Department of Microbiology
Vaagdevi Degree and PG College
Hanamkonda, Warangal
Telangana State, India

Dr. K. Srisailam

Principal
University College of Pharmaceutical Sciences
Shatavahana University
Karimnagar
Telangana State, India

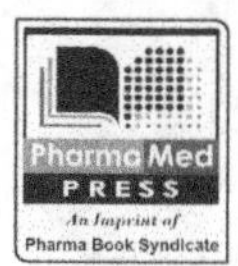

PharmaMed Press
An imprint of Pharma Book Syndicate
A unit of BSP Books Pvt. Ltd.
4-4-309/316, Giriraj Lane,
Sultan Bazar, Hyderabad - 500 095.

Pharmaceutical Microbiology: A Laboratory Manual
by G. Shyam Prasad and K. Srisailam

Published by

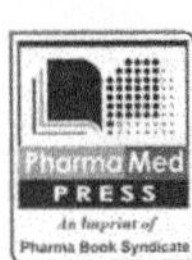

PharmaMed Press

An imprint of Pharma Book Syndicate

A unit of BSP Books Pvt. Ltd.

4-4-309/316, Giriraj Lane, Sultan Bazar, Hyderabad - 500 095.
Phone: 040-23445688, 23445600; Fax: 91+40-23445611
E-mail: info@pharmamedpress.com
www.pharmamedpress.com/pharmamedpress.net

ISBN: 978-93-88305-02-0 (Hardback)

This book is Dedicated to

Prof. (Dr). G. Upender
Father of **Dr. G. Shyam Prasad**

PREFACE

Pharmaceutical Microbiology is an applied branch of Microbiology which deals with the study of microorganisms associated with manufacturing and quality control of pharmaceutical products.

The present book *"Pharmaceutical Microbiology: A Laboratory Manual"* meets the syllabus designed by the Pharmacy Council of India and is written with a holistic approach encompassing various topics of Experimental Pharmaceutical Microbiology. This manual covers nearly 50 experiments based on General and Pharmaceutical Microbiology which would serve as a guide to B-pharmacy students of all the Indian Universities. The main aim of writing this book is to cover theoretical and experimental parts of all the topics included in the curriculum for Experimental Pharmaceutical Microbiology given in the revised syllabus of B.Pharm students. The various concepts and phenomenon have been explained in simple terms with the help of appropriate diagrams.

The experimental methods are tailor made to meet the modest facilities available in many of the colleges and universities within the country.

The authors appreciate all constructive suggestions and criticism for improvement of this book.

G. Shyam Prasad

K. Srisailam

ACKNOWLEDGEMENTS

We wish to extend our special thanks to **Prof. S. M. Reddy** and **Prof. S. Girisham,** Department of Microbiology, Kakatiya University, Warangal and **Prof. B. Sashidhar Rao**, and **Dr. Karuna Rupula**, Department of Biochemistry, Osmania University, Hyderabad for their constant support and encouragement.

Above all, we are thankful to **G. Preethi** W/o G. Shyam Prasad and **E. Sujatha**, W/o K. Srisailam, for their patience and extending support while writing this book.

Finally, we would like to thank **G. Kamala, G. Ram Prasad, G. Akshaya Priya, G. Snithik, Dr. B. Devi, Dr. R. Chandra Mohan Rao**. They all kept us going and this book wouldn't have been possible without them.

G. Shyam Prasad

K. Srisailam

CONTENTS

Techniques for Isolation of Pure Culture from Mixed Culture

Staining Techniques of Microorganisms

Biochemical Tests for Identification of Bacteria

Bacterial Motility

MICROBIOLOGY LABORATORY:
BASIC RULES AND REQUIREMENTS

1

Pharmaceutical Microbiology and Basic Rules of Laboratory

Pharmaceutical Microbiology

Microbiology is a branch of biology which deals with the study of very minute living organisms such as bacteria, protozoa, fungi and similar organisms that can't be seen with the naked eye. Pharmaceutical microbiology is an applied branch of microbiology which is responsible for the production of antibiotics, enzymes, vaccines, vitamins and other pharmaceutical substances. It also deals with microorganisms which contaminate pharmaceutical products, minimizing the number of microorganisms in a process environment, excluding microorganisms and microbial by-products like exotoxin and endotoxin from water and other starting materials. It ensures that medications do not contain harmful levels of microbes- such as bacteria, yeast and molds. It mainly focuses on the manufacturing techniques, process controls, and finished product attributes that limit the harmful effects of microorganisms on the drug product. Pharmaceutical products can save lives and bring back the health of patients, but what if these products are contaminated? The presence of a microbial contaminant in pharmaceutical products can reduce or even inactivate the therapeutic activity of the products and has the potential to adversely affect patients taking the medicines. The contaminating microorganisms may cause spoilage of the product with loss of its therapeutic properties and, if they are pathogenic, serious infections can arise. Furthermore, the presence of bad bugs in pharmaceutical products can lead to costly product recalls resulting in financial and image losses, loss of product sales, decreased customer confidence, and in many cases, legal proceedings.

Thus, it is important to know the microbial content of all drugs and medicines, whether they are sterile or non-sterile and to implement strict microbial controls to ensure that the final products are consistent, safe, effective and predictable.

A. Microbiology Lab Practices and Safety Rules

1. Leave your footwear in the rack provided before entering microbiology lab and wear lab footwear available at the entrance of the lab.

2. Familiarize yourself with the location of instruments and safety equipment in the lab (e.g., eye-wash station, first aid kit etc)

3. Wash your hands with disinfectant soap when you arrive at the lab and wear lab coat available inside the rack provided at the entrance of the lab.

4. Absolutely do not eat drinks or smoke in the laboratory. Even do not put anything in mouth such as pencils, pens, labels, or fingers. Do not store food in areas where microorganisms are stored.

5. Disinfect work areas before and after use with 70% ethanol or propanol.

6. Ensure that all the instruments viz. refrigerator, incubator, oven, laminar air flow, autoclave are in proper working conditions. And also check for availability of chemicals before starting the work.

7. Long hair should be tied back to minimize contamination of cultures and fire hazards

8. Protect yourself from exposure to eyes and skin to UV light by wearing goggles and clothing respectively.

9. All cultures and prepared solutions should be labeled or marked clearly with the date of preparation.

10. Before using any microbial culture ensure that you are using the right culture.

11. Wear gloves and mask when working with pathogenic microbial cultures.

12. Aseptic conditions should be strictly followed at all times to avoid contamination.

13. If any culture has to be used, please check for purity and see that further stock of culture is available for future work.

14. Never pipette out broth cultures or bacterial suspensions in saline, with the mouth.

15. Always keep culture tubes in upright position in a rack or basket

16. If live culture is spilled, cover the area with a disinfectant for 15min and then clean with 70% isopropyl alcohol or ethanol.

17. Label all the culture plates, tubes properly before starting an experiment.

18. Inoculating loops and needles should be flame sterilized in a Bunsen burner before you laying them down after inoculation.

19. Wear disposable gloves when working with potentially infectious microbes or samples. If you are working with a sample that may contain a pathogen, then be extremely careful to use a good bacteriological technique.

20. Turn off Bunsen burners when not in use. Long hair must be restrained if Bunsen burners are in use.

21. Dispose off all used agar and broth cultures after incubation period in a biohazard bag and autoclave it before discarding in the regular trash. Do not pour anything down the sink.

22. In the event of personal injuries such as cuts or burns inform your instructor immediately as bacteria enter open wounds

23. Dispose of broken glass in the broken glass container.

24. Replace caps on reagents, solution bottles, and bacterial cultures. Do not open Petri dishes with cultures in the lab unless absolutely necessary.

25. Always clean microscope before and after use. Clean lenses with lens paper.

26. Decontaminate laboratory equipment and work surfaces with an appropriate disinfectant on a routine basis, and especially after spills, splashes, or other contamination.

27. Wash your hands and place the apron and footwear at the place provided before leaving the lab.

2

Basic Requirements of Microbiology Laboratory

A. Instruments
1. Microscope
2. Autoclave
3. Hot air oven
4. Incubator
5. BOD Incubator
6. Digital balance
7. pH meter
8. Laminar air flow
9. Inoculation loops
10. Inoculation needles
11. Bunsen burner
12. Refrigerator
13. Centrifuge
14. Water bath
15. Distillation unit
16. Colony counter
17. Centrifuge
18. Cyclomixer
19. Spectrophotometer

B. Glassware
1. Petri plates
2. Test tubes/culture tubes
3. Glass rods
4. Pasteur pipette
5. Erlenmeyer conical flasks
6. Measuring cylinders
7. Spreader
8. Micropipette
9. Burettes

C. Miscellaneous
1. Test tube rack
2. Stains and staining racks
3. Cotton/ Cotton plugs
4. Glass markers
5. Scissors
6. Rubber bands
7. Forceps

INSTRUMENTATION

Microscope

A microscope (microscope: micro - small scope - look) is an optical instrument consisting of a lens or combination of lenses for making enlarged images of minute objects that are too small to be seen by naked eye. A compound microscope has optical and mechanical portions.

I. Optical Portion:

The optical portion has two types of lenses for greater magnification and consists of the ocular and objective lens. The magnification is due to eyepiece and the objective lens.

a. The ocular lens (eyepiece) that one looks into

The ocular lens or the eyepiece is the lens present at the top that you look through. The image magnified by the objective lens is further magnified by the ocular lens. The ocular lenses are usually 10X, 15X etc.

b. The objective lens or the lens closest to the object.

The objective lens consists of several lenses to magnify an object and project a larger image. Most of the compound microscopes have three objective lens.

i.   **Low power**: It has a focal length of 16mm and ten times the original. Hence marked as 10X. This lens when coupled with a 10X eyepiece the total magnification becomes 100X (10X times 10X).

ii. **High power**: It has the focal length of 40mm and forty times the original, hence marked as 40X. This lens when coupled with a 10X eyepiece the total magnification becomes 400X (40X times 10X).

iii. **Oil immersion**: It has a focal length of 18mm and gives a magnification hundred times the original and is marked 100X.

This lens when coupled with a 10X eyepiece the total magnification becomes 1000X (100X times 10X).

> **Total magnification = Magnifying power of objective ×
> Magnifying power of eye piece**

II. Mechanical Portion: The non- optical portion (mechanical portion) consists of the following parts

   a. **Body Tube**: A hollow tube which connects eyepiece to the objective lens through which light travels from the objective to the ocular.

   b. **Arm**: C-shaped arm is present between the foot and body tube. It is meant for the support of the body tube.

   c. **Coarse and fine adjustment knobs**: The coarse adjustment knob is located on the arm of the microscope which moves the stage up and down to bring the specimen into focus.

   d. **Fine adjustment knob**: This is also located on the arm and is used to bring the specimen into sharp focus.

   e. **Revolving Nose piece:** It is provided with several objective lenses of varying magnification and numerical aperture.

   f. **Stage:** This is the horizontal surface upon which the slide is placed. The slide is held in place by spring loaded clips and moved around the stage by turning the geared knobs on the stage.

      i. **Devices for controlling light**: Optimum amount of light should be provided and the microscopes are provided with light just below the stage. The sources of light are usually sun or an electric bulb.

      ii. **Condenser**: It is located immediately under the stage and condenses the irregular beams of light into the specimen.

      iii. **Mirror:** It can be adjusted in different planes to reflect light from the sources. The mirrors may be with a plane or concave surface. A plane surface is used when the rays are parallel i.e. when the source is very distant. The concave surface is used when the rays are from a nearby source as the electric bulb.

   iv. **Diaphragm:** It is a strong rotating disk under the stage. The diaphragm has different sized holes and is used to vary the intensity and size of the cone of light that is projected upwards into the specimen.

  g. **Base:** A broad U shaped or horse-shoe shaped basal foot is present supporting the microscope (base)

Focusing a microscope:

1. Start with the lowest power objective lens first and while looking from the side, crank the lens down as close to the specimen as possible without touching it.

2. Adjust the mirrors employing the appropriate surface

3. The condenser is adjusted to allow optimum light

4. Now looking through the eyepiece focus upward only until the image is sharp.

5. Once the image is sharp with the low power lens, simply click in the next power lens and do minor adjustments with the focus knob.

6. Continue with subsequent objective lenses and fine focus each time.

Technique and objective of oil immersion:

a. After focusing the clear image of the object under low power objective, rotate the nose piece and bring the oil immersion objective into its position.

b. A drop of sterile mineral oil is placed on the object and the body tube lowered until the objective touches the oil surface and care should be taken that the objective does not touch the specimen. Using a little coarse adjustment and fine adjustment the object is brought into sharp focus. After the examination, the oil adhering to the surface of the lens of objective is removed using a lens paper.

c. The prime objective of oil immersion is to use the oil of the same refractive index as that of glass such that the rays of light do not get scattered or disturbed. The dust particles if present may provide errors in the examination.

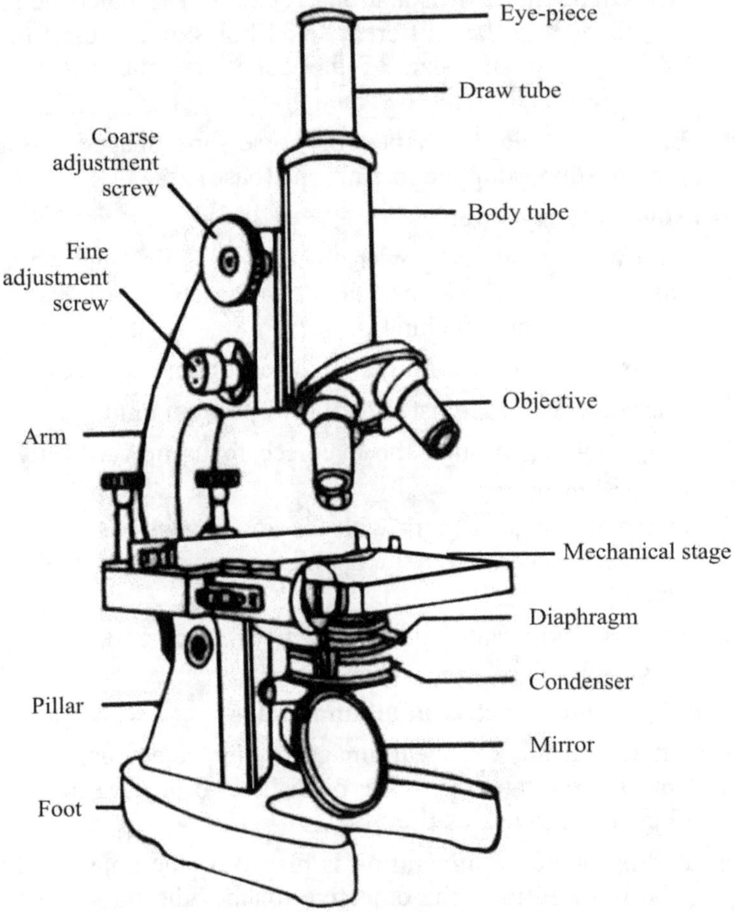

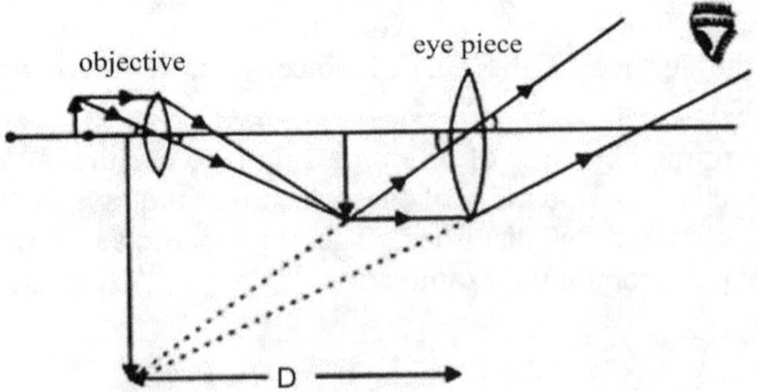

A compound microscope

Precautions:

a. Never carry the microscope with one hand

b. The objective and the eyepiece are cleaned and kept dry

c. Fix the slide in proper position on the stage

d. The oil adhering to the surface of objective lens is removed using a lens paper.

e. Use proper side of the mirror for proper illumination.

f. On completion of work, microscope should be cleaned and kept away from moisture and dust.

g. First focus carefully on low power objective and later turn to high power.

Theoretical Principles of Microscopy:

1. **Magnification:**

   Enlargement or magnification of a specimen is the function of a two-lens system; the ocular lens is found in the eyepiece, and the objective lens is situated in a revolving nose-piece. These lenses are separated by the body tube. The objective lens is nearer the specimen and magnifies it, producing the real image that is projected up into the focal plane and then magnified by the ocular lens to produce the final image.

Objective lens	Ocular lens	Total magnification
Lower power 10X	10X	100X
High power 40X	10C	400X
Oil Immersion 100X	10X	1000X

2. **Resolving power or resolution:**

   Unlimited magnification is not possible by merely increasing the magnifying power of the lenses because lenses are limited by a property called resolving power. Resolving power is the ability of a lens to distinguish two very small and closely placed adjacent objects as separate entities. When a lens cannot discriminate, that is, when the two objects appear as one, it has lost resolution. Increased magnification will not rectify the loss, and will, in fact, blur the object. The resolving power of a lens is dependent on the wavelength of light used and the numerical aperture, which is a characteristic of each lens.

$$\text{Resolving power} = \frac{\text{Wavelength of light}}{(\text{Numerical aperture})1}$$

3. **Numerical aperture:**

   Numerical aperture is light gathering capabilities of a lens. The better the light gathering property of the lens, the better the resolution. The Numerical aperture of the condenser is as important as the numerical aperture of the objective lens in determining resolution. It is for this reason that the closure of the condenser diaphragm results in a loss of resolution.

4. **Refractive index:**

   The refractive index determines how much the path of light is bent or refracted when passing from one medium to another. The imaging medium for microscopy is air which has refractive index lower than glass, so when light is passed from air to glass slide it is bent or refracted. To compensate the refracted light, mineral oil is used which has same refractive index as glass.

5. **Illumination:**

   For efficient magnification and resolving power effective illumination is required. Since the intensity of daylight is an uncontrolled variable, artificial light from a tungsten lamp is the most commonly used light source for microscopy. The condenser should be used for proper illumination and it should be closed when oil immersion objective is used.

4

Autoclave

An Autoclave is the most essential instrument used in microbiology laboratory for sterilization. It is based on the principle that saturated steam under pressure kills microorganisms. The water boils at 100°C and the steam accumulates in a closed container resulting in an increase in pressure. It is not the pressure that kills the organisms but the high temperature of the steam. The boiling point of water at 15psi pressure is 121°C. Most of the organisms are killed at 121°C (15psi) in 15 minutes including the heat-resistant spore-formers. Steam temperature increases with increase in steam pressure. The autoclave is used for sterilization of media both solid and liquid, heat stable liquids, heat resistant instruments glassware and rubber products. It is also used to sterilize glassware when required.

Design of autoclave

An autoclave is a double –walled metallic vessel. The body is usually made up of steel or aluminium. The lid is provided with a pressure guage for recording the pressure, steam cock (exhaust value) for air exhaustation, a safety value to avoid explosions. Both vertical and horizontal types of autoclaves are available, but for routine laboratory use vertical types are commonly used.

Operation:

1. In standard vertical autoclave, sufficient quantity of distilled water is added at the bottom of the autoclave till the mark so that the heating coil dips completely.

2. The objects to be sterilized are wrapped properly in a paper or aluminium foil and loaded in the basket provided and placed at the bottom of the autoclave.

3. Objects are loaded in such a way that facilitates the steam to be directly in contact with the surface.

4. Now place the lid of the autoclave and tighten the opposite screws provided.

5. Switch on the autoclave by keeping the steam release valve open so that air inside the autoclave is allowed to escape completely through this valve.

6. Close the valve when water vapor is seen to escape through it.

7. Temperature and pressure inside goes on increasing. The pressure increase is observed in the pressure gauge.

8. Usually, sterilization is done at 121 °C (a pressure of 15 pounds per square inch i.e. 15 psi) for 15 minutes.

9. The required time is considered from the point, when the required temperature-pressure is attained. Once required temperature-pressure is attained, it is maintained.

10. After the specified time (15 minutes), switch off the autoclave and open slightly the steam release valve. If fully opened immediately, due to sudden fall in pressure, liquids may spill out from the containers.

11. Autoclave lid is opened only after the pressure drops back to normal atmospheric pressure (0 psi).

12. Unload the hot sterilized materials by holding them with a piece of clean cloth or asbestos- coated hand gloves.

13. Transfer the sterilized material immediately to laminar air flow.

Relationship between pressure and temperature in an autoclave:

Pressure in pounds per Square inch (psi)	Temperature in °C
5	109
10	115.6
15	121.0
20	126.0
25	130

Precautions:

1. The water level inside the autoclave should be well above the heating coil.

2. If water is less, the bottom of the autoclave gets dried during heating and burns the heating coil. On the other hand, if there is too much water, it takes a long time to reach the required temperature.

3. Always tighten the opposite screw while closing the lid on all sides.

4. The air in the chamber of autoclave must be completely replaced by pure steam. Keep open the steam outlet until pure steam starts going out.

5. The autoclave should never be opened, when there is pressure inside.

6. The required 15 psi pressure must be maintained constantly for 15 minutes

7. Overcooking of the medium will change the composition of the medium and may not support microbial growth, Agar may also lose the gelling (solidifying) property

8. Do not open the lid until the pressure gauge shows zero.

9. The Autoclave should get validated periodically.

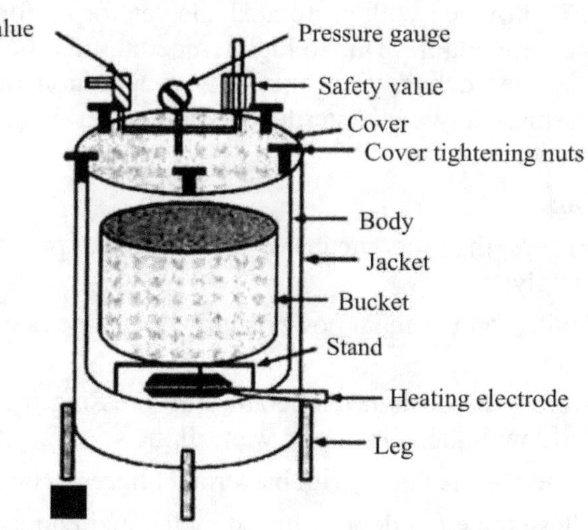

A Schematic diagram of laboratory autoclave

5

Incubator

An incubator is a double walled jacket insulated to check heat conduction and provided with double doors. The inner door is made of glass so as to view the contents of the incubator without disturbing temperature conditions of the cabinet. An incubator consisting of a heating element at the bottom, a thermostat, temperature probe and devices for regulating the temperature. A proper temperature recording thermometer is provided by inserting from the top to record the temperature. An incubator provides controlled, contaminant free environment for incubating, maintaining the cultures at constant desired temperature at or above the ambient temperature. An ideal temperature for most of the bacteria is 35±2°C. However, the desired temperature can be adjusted with a thermostat. It is designed in such a way to maintain the temperature below 80°C. The incubator is provided with perforated shelves for uniform maintenance of the desired temperature. Due to high temperature in the incubator, there is a possibility for dehydration and slow evaporation of culture medium. Hence, a small tray with sterile distilled water is provided inside the incubator at the bottom.

Operation:

1. Ensure that the incubator is connected properly to the power supply.
2. Switch on the main power supply and check power indicator light is on.
3. Adjust the desired temperature by pressing the set knob and soft keys with the help of and wait till the set temperature is reached.
4. Load the incubator with bacterial cultures to be incubated.
5. Close the glass door followed by the main door.

Precautions:

1. Do not place incubator at the entrance of the lab
2. Open the door of the incubator only when needed
3. Do not overload the incubator
4. Cotton plugs should be pushed inside the neck of the test tube to prevent evaporation of the medium.
5. Monitor the temperature of incubator daily to ensure proper working
6. Switch off the incubator when not in use.
7. Clean the metallic surfaces (racks, floor, walls and doors) with 70% ethanol after every experiment.
8. Ensure that the sterile distilled water is available in the tray provided at the bottom of the incubator.

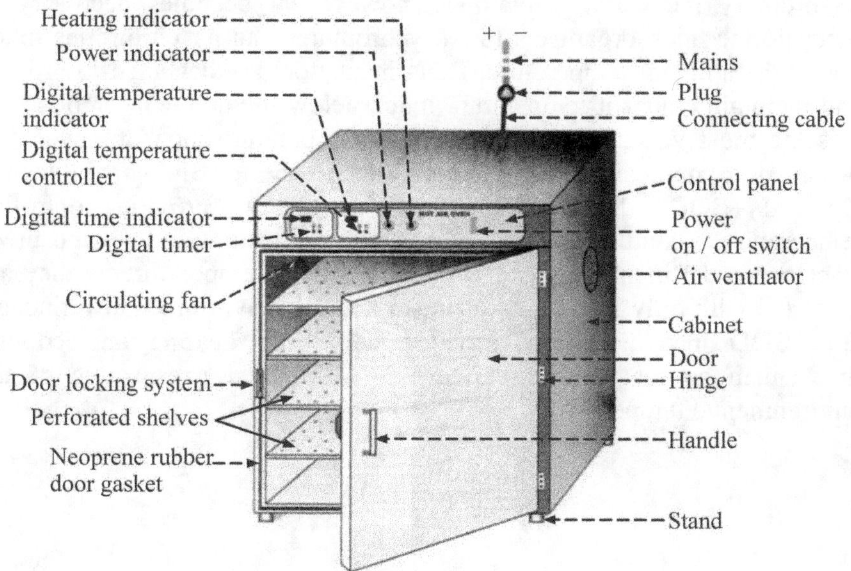

Bacteriological Incubator

Biological Oxygen Demand Incubator (BOD)
(Low Temperature Incubator)

Some microbes are to be grown at lower temperatures for specific purposes. The BOD incubator also is known as low temperature incubators because, they are designed with temperatures range from 5°C to as high as 60°C with cooling and heating function under one unit. The constant desired temperature is set by rotating the knob of the thermostat. Exact required temperature is obtained, by rotating the knob finely by trial and error and noting the temperature on the thermometer fixed on the incubator. Most of the modern BOD incubators are programmable, which do not need trial and error temperature setting. Here, the operator sets the desired temperature and the required period of time. The incubator automatically maintains accordingly.

A temperature less than ambient temperature cannot be maintained in an ordinary incubator. Sometimes, however, it becomes necessary to incubate the microorganisms like psychrophiles and psychrotrophs much below the ambient temperature. BOD incubators are designed to provide and maintain constant temperature much below the ambient temperature. It is the most versatile and reliable low temperature incubator which is designed to maintain at or at 20°C, necessary for Biological Oxygen Demand (BOD) determination. BOD incubators provide controlled temperature conditions for accelerated tests and exposures. Bacteriological incubators can maintain only set temperature as they are provided with only heating mechanism and has environmental influence. But, BOD incubators are provided with both heating and cooling mechanism so that set temperature is maintained irrespective of the environmental temperature.

Hot Air Oven

Hot air oven is an electrical device which uses dry heat for sterilization. It was originally developed by Pasteur. Hot air oven accomplishes sterilization by dry heat or dry air. Dry heat removes water from microorganisms and all macromolecules lose their structure and ability to function. The killing effect of dry heat is due to denaturation of proteins, oxidative damage and elevated levels of electrolytes. Dry heat destroys bacterial endotoxins (or pyrogens) which are difficult to eliminate by other means. The benefit of dry heat includes good penetrability and non-corrosive nature which makes it applicable for sterilization and it will not leave any chemical residue. Hot air oven suits to various applications like drying and sterilization.

Items that are not to be sterilized in a hot air oven include:

- Surgical dressings
- Rubber items, or plastic material
- Liquid substances, such as prepared media and saline solutions cannot be sterilized in oven, as they lose water due to evaporation.

Items that can be sterilized in a hot air oven include:

- Glassware (Petri dishes, flasks, pipettes, and test tubes)
- Powders (starch, zinc oxide, and sulfadiazine)
- Metal equipment (scalpels, scissors, and blades)
- It is also used for sterilizing non-aqueous thermostable liquids and thermostable powders.

Construction of Oven

An oven consists of an insulated, heat proof cabinet which maintains a desired constant temperature with the help of electric heating mechanism and a thermostat-control, using which the required constant temperature can be obtained by trial and error but the reading is approximate and the exact temperature is read by introducing a thermometer into the oven or on a built-in L-shaped thermometer. The oven is also fitted with a fan to keep the hot air circulating at a constant temperature. Shelves inside the oven are perforated to facilitate the free circulation of air. Ovens are most commonly used for sterilization of glassware like Petri plates, test tubes, pipettes, metal instruments that can withstand prolonged heat exposure. Normally, all the routine glassware is sterilized by keeping at 160°C for 2 hours. A schedule of time and temperature for sterilization with dry air is presented in table

Temperature °C	Sterilization time (in minutes)
120	480
140	180
150	150
160	120
170	60
180	20

Procedure:

1. Glassware to be sterilized is washed properly and air dried.

2. Materials are first wrapped or enclosed in containers of steel or aluminum.

3. Later, they are arranged inside the oven to ensure uninterrupted air flow.

4. The power is switched on and allowed to run for the desired time as shown in table.

5. Then the power is switched off and the temperature is allowed to fall to 40°C, prior to removal of sterilized material.

6. In a modern oven, there is a digital temperature display and automatic temperature controller to set the desired temperature easily and the oven switches off automatically after the set time.

7. The oven door is opened, only after its temperature comes down near to room temperature. Otherwise, cold air may rush in and crack the glassware.

Precautions:

1. Dry glassware completely before loading into hot air oven.

2. Wrap glassware in kraft papers. Do not overload the oven. Overloading alters heat convection and increases the time required to sterilize.

3. Allow free circulation of air between the materials.

4. The article and substances which are to be sterilized should not be placed on the floor of the oven as it receives direct heat and becomes much hotter.

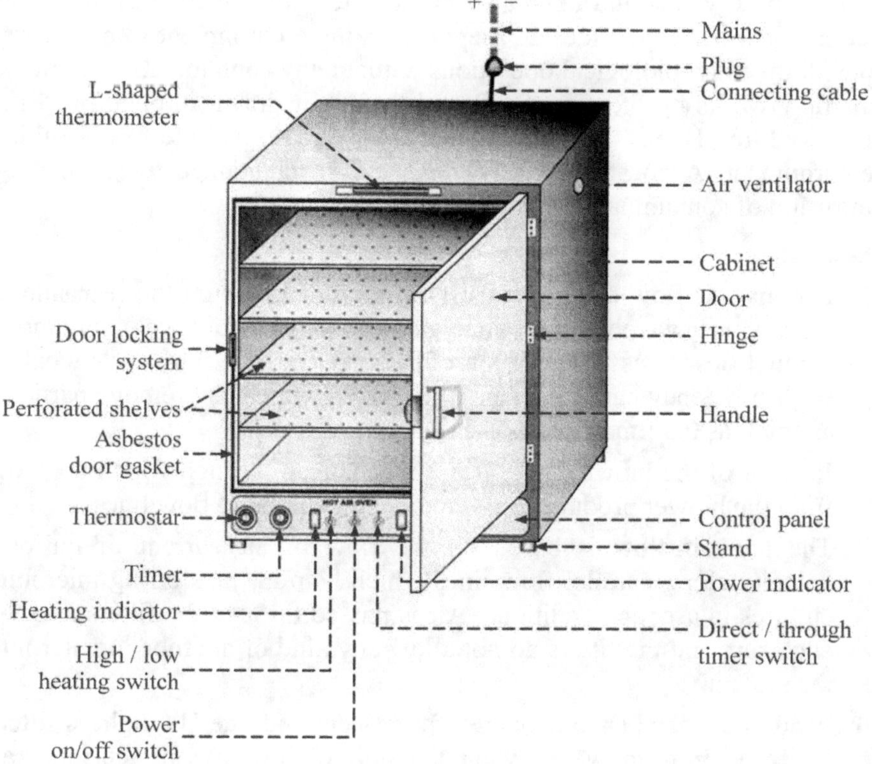

Hot air Oven

Laminar Air Flow

A laminar air flow cabinet is a carefully enclosed bench designed to control both viable and nonviable particulate contamination during clean assembly work. It provides an aseptic working environment so as to carry out all the microbiological operations without any contamination. Laminar air flow works by the use of inflow laminar air drawn through pre filter followed by HEPA filter designed to create a particle-free working environment. A constant positive pressure is maintained to prevent the intrusion of contaminated room air.

Design:

1. Laminar air flow cabinet consists of an air blower on the rear side of the chamber which can produce air flow with uniform velocity among parallel flow lines. There is a prefilter and a special filter system called High-efficiency particulate air filter HEPA which can remove particles as small as 0.3 μm.

2. In front of the blower there lies a mechanism through which air blow from the blower produces air velocity along parallel flow lines.

3. The laminar flow is based on the flow of air current of uniform velocity along parallel flow lines which help in transferring microbial cultures in aseptic conditions. Air is passed through the filters into the enclosure and the filters do not allow any kind of microbe to enter into the system.

4. Inside the chamber, one or two fluorescent and one UV light is fitted. Due to uniform velocity and parallel flow of air current, all microbiological operations like transfer of cultures, pouring of media, platting, purifications etc. can be carried out without any contamination.

5. Both horizontal and vertical laminar air flow cabinets are available.

Operation:

1. Switch on the UV light and air flow 30mins before starting the work so as to decontaminate the chamber.

2. Put off the UV light after 30 minutes and switch on the fluorescent lights keeping flow on.

3. Open the front door of the laminar air flow cabin, not more than 10 inches and wear sterilized powder free hand gloves to both the hands.

4. Spray down the alcohol to gloves and rub both the hands so as to free the hands with microbes.

5. Disinfect the entire work area of laminar airflow with 70% alcohol using sterilized smooth cloth.

6. All operations inside the cabinet should be carried out in the flame zone of the Bunsen burner.

7. After completion of testing, clean the working table with 70% alcohol.

8. Switch off the fluorescent lights and airflow and switch on the UV light for 30 minutes.

9. Switch off the UV light after 30 minutes.

Precautions:

1. Do not enter LAF room with regular footwear.

2. Wash hands with detergent or soap before entering LAF room.

3. Check daily and ensure that the manometer reading on LAF is as per the specified limits.

4. Don't look directly into UV light, wear goggles.

5. All objects in the hood should be placed towards the back but not laid across the back wall as blocking the baffles reduces airflow.

6. After finishing the work, clean the platform with 70% alcohol.

7. Switch on the UV light and keep for 30 minutes after completion of the work.

8. If a spill occurs, clean immediately with a disinfectant.

9. Do not switch on the UV light during working period.

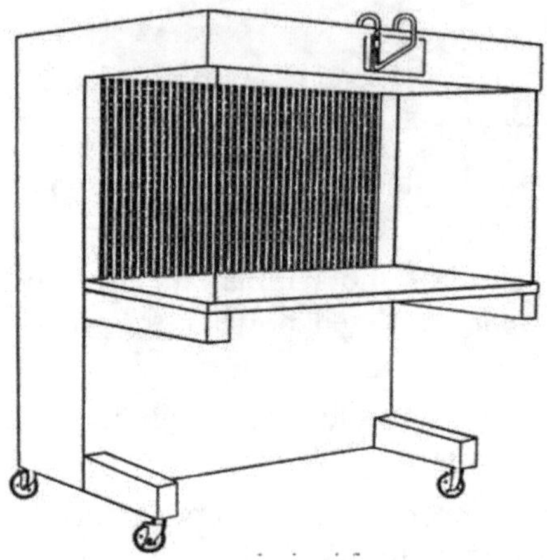

Laminar air flow

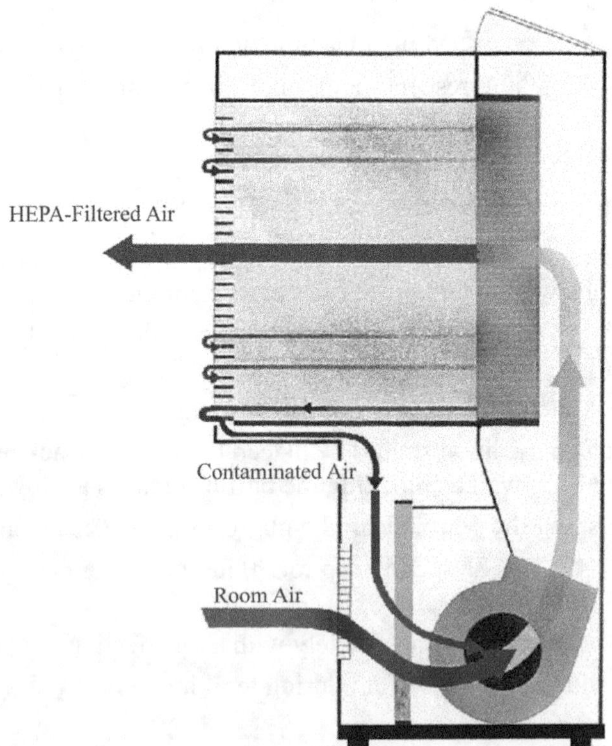

Working of laminar air flow

8

pH Meter

The pH meter is used to determine acidity or alkalinity of an unknown solution. The acidity or alkalinity of a solution is determined by the relative number of hydrogen ions (H+) or hydroxyl ions (OH) present. Acidic solutions have a higher relative number of hydrogen ions; whereas alkaline solutions have a higher relative number of hydroxyl ions. In microbiological laboratory pH meter is used for measuring or adjusting the pH of various media used in the cultivation of and testing of biochemical activities of microorganisms as maintaining of pH is an important parameter for the growth of any organism.

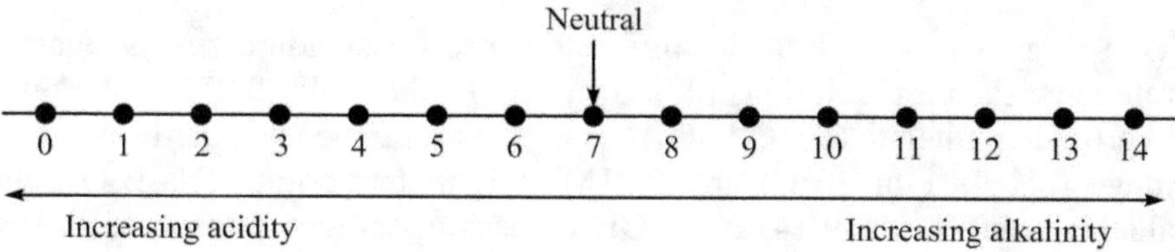

pH scale

Construction and working of pH meter:

1. Two main parts of a pH meter are an electrode (Probe) which is a special measuring rod like structure and an analyzer or display to which probe is connected.

2. At the bottom of the electrode, there is a bulb which is a very sensitive part.

3. Electrode contains a silver alloy wire submerged in a neutral solution (pH 7.0) of potassium chloride. In addition to the glass electrode, the pH meter also consists of another electrode called the reference electrode which also has a silver alloy wire submerged in neutral potassium chloride solution located in an outer glass tube.

4. When the electrode is dipped in a test solution and if the hydrogen ion concentration inside the electrode differs from hydrogen ion concentration of test solution a measurable potential difference forms.

5. The pH value is calculated from the potential difference between the reference electrode and the test solution.

   a. If the hydrogen ion concentration is less inside the electrode than hydrogen ion concentration of test solution, the measured solution is acidic i.e., the pH value is less than 7.0.

   b. If the hydrogen ion concentration is more inside the electrode than hydrogen ion concentration of test solution, then the measured solution is alkaline i.e., the pH value is greater than 7.0.

   c. If the hydrogen ion concentration is identical on both sides no potential difference forms and the measured solution's pH is neutral with pH value 7.0.

Calibration of pH meter:

The pH meter is calibrated daily before use by standardizing it against reference standard solutions of known pH. Traditionally 0.05M potassium hydroxide phthalate ($KHC_8H_4O_4$) is used as reference standard for acidic range (pH 4.01 at 30°C) and 0.01M sodium tetraborate ($Na_2B_4O_7$) for alkaline range (pH 9.14 at 30°C). Potassium-sodium phosphate buffer (0.05M is used as reference standard for neutral pH (pH 6.85 at 30°C).

Maintenance of electrode:

1. Electrode should be filled with saturated potassium chloride solution up to the height of about 1cm below the filling hole.

2. Shake the electrode gently to ensure that the internal buffer covers the whole membrane and no air bubbles are present.

3. Wash off any salt film present outside the electrode using distilled water.

4. Clean the electrode with the distilled water after every use.

5. Always keep the electrode dipped in distilled water when not in use.

Precautions:

1. pH meter should be calibrated before each measurement.
2. Calibration should be performed with at least two fresh standard buffer solutions.
3. Never touch the bulb as it is a sensitive part of the probe.
4. Soak the electrode in distilled water for the overnight before using for the first time.

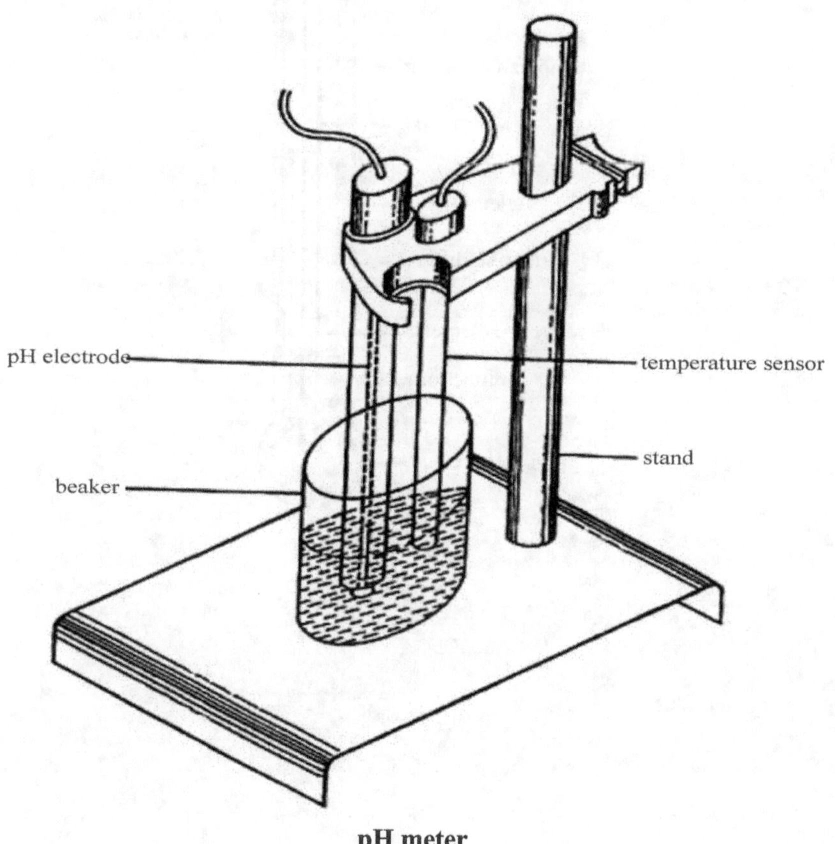

pH meter

refill opening
temperature sensor
Silver (AgCl) wire
electrolyte
internal buffer
reference element
junction
glass membrance

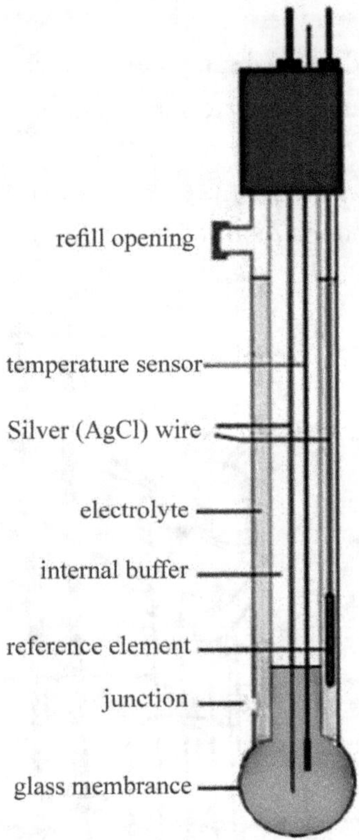

Electrode

9

Spectrophotometer

A spectrophotometer is an instrument that measures the amount of light absorbed by a substance. Every chemical compound absorbs, transmits, or reflects light over a certain range of wavelength. Spectrophotometry is a measurement of how much a chemical substance absorbs or transmits light after it passes through the sample solution. UV-visible spectrophotometer uses light over the ultraviolet range (185 - 400 nm) and visible range (400 - 700 nm) of electromagnetic radiation spectrum.

A spectrophotometer, in general consists of two devices; a spectrometer and a photometer. A spectrometer is a device that produces, typically disperses and measures light. A photometer indicates the photoelectric detector that measures the intensity of light.

- **Spectrometer**: It produces a desired range of wavelength of light. First, a collimator (lens) transmits a straight beam of light (photons) that passes through a monochromator (prism) to split it into several component wavelengths (spectrum). Then a wavelength selector (slit) transmits only the desired wavelengths.

- **Photometer**: After the desired range of wavelength of light passes through the solution of a sample in the cuvette, the photometer detects the photons that are absorbed and then sends a signal to a digital display.

Transmittance (T): It is a measure of the fraction of light that passes through the sample. It is the ratio between I and I_0

$$T = \frac{I}{I_0}$$

The percentage transmittance (%T) = %T = T × 100

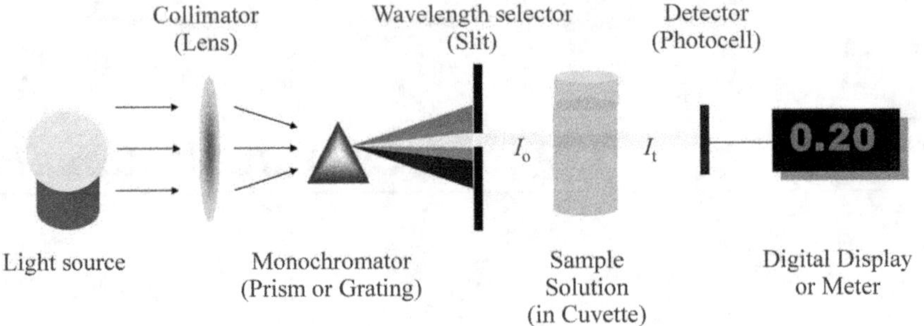

Components of a spectrophotometer

I_0 = intensity of incident light I_t = Intensity of transmitted light

Absorbance (A): is the amount of light absorbed by the sample

$$A = -\log T = -\log \frac{I}{I_0}$$

The absorbance in terms of percentage transmittance:

$$A = 2 - \log (\%T)$$

Beer-Lambert's law: It is the fundamental law on which quantitative measurements in colorimetry and spectrometry are based. This law states that the amount of incident radiation absorbed or transmitted by a solution is proportional to the total concentration of absorbing molecules present in the light path.

$$A = \epsilon l\, c$$

Where

A = absorbance

ϵ = Molar absorption coefficient

l = Length of light path through the sample or thickness of the sample cell

c = concentration of the absorbing substance in the sample

10

Colony Counter

Digital Colony counter is designed for quick and accurate counting of bacterial and mold colonies on the surface of Petri dishes. This is an indispensable benchtop tool for the busy microbiologist. Colony counter is used to estimate a liquid cultures density of microorganisms by counting individual colonies on the agar surface.

Operating Procedure:

1. Connect the instrument to the main power supply.
2. Switch on the instrument.
3. Place the Petridish containing bacterial colonies in the space provided.
4. The instrument is provided with 100mm diameter magnifying lens and auto pen marker.
5. Take the auto-marker pen and mark each colony by pressing the pen tip and the Digital counter will start counting sequentially.
6. The counter can be set to zero by pressing the centre push button.
7. Counting can also be done manually without using pen marker by pressing the push button provided at right hand side of the panel.
8. The instrument displays four-digit counter with beep sound for each counting.

Precautions:

1. Disinfect hands with 70% IPA.
2. Do not open the lid of Petri plate while counting colonies.
3. Press the marker pen on Petri plates till the audio buzzer indicates beep sound.

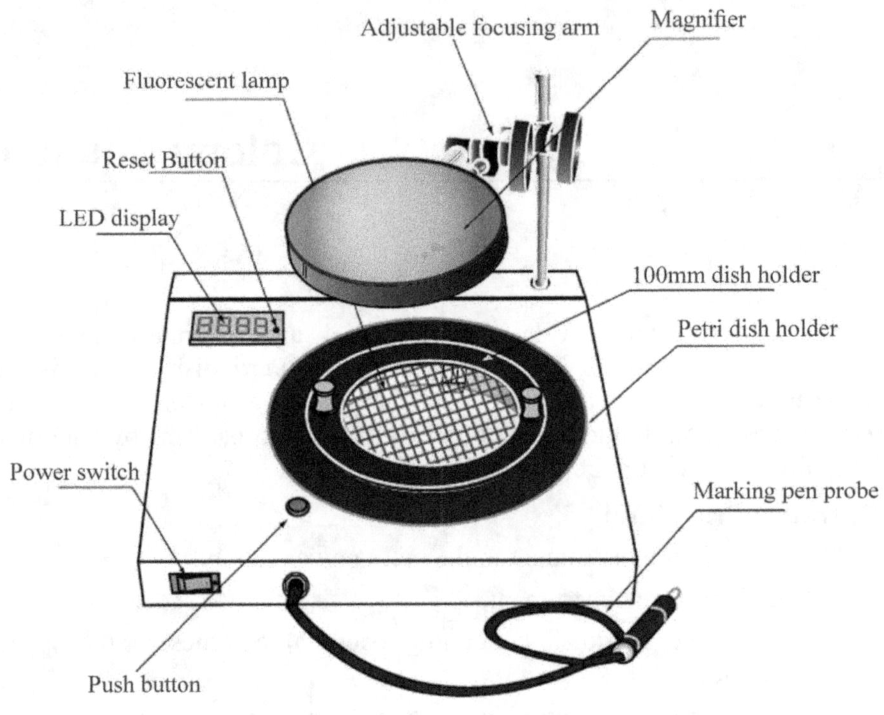

Colony counter

PREPARATION OF CULTURE MEDIA, STERILIZATION AND CULTURE METHODS

11

Preparation and Sterilization of Media

Microbial culture media are nutrient preparation used in laboratories to grow microorganisms whose survival, growth and division depends on the availability of nutrients and a favorable environment. For the successful cultivation of a given microorganism, it is necessary to understand its nutritional requirements and supply the essential nutrients in the proper form and proportion in a culture medium. Not all bacteria grow optimally on the same kind of medium, nor do all bacteria grow optimally at the same temperature or pH. There are different types of media available.

a. Preparation of nutrient broth:

Requirements:

Peptone

Beef extract

Distilled water

pH meter

Autoclave

Test tubes

HCl-1N

NaOH-IN

Laminar air flow

Weighing balance

Procedure:

1. Weigh required amount of media ingredients as per media composition and transfer into a clean conical flask.

2. Add the desired amount of distilled water and mix properly with glass rod so that all the ingredients are mixed properly.

3.   Check the pH of the medium and adjust if required to the desired to support luxuriant growth of experimental microbes.

4.   Plug the mouth of the conical flask with cotton.

5.   Cover the mouth of the cotton plugs with aluminium foil or a paper and bind with a rubber band.

6.   Later, transfer the media containing conical flask/tubes to the autoclave and sterilize at 121°C for 15-minutes at 15 lbs pressure.

7.   After autoclaving, allow media to cool and incubate a portion of media at 37°C for 24-48 h in an incubator to check for any bacterial growth and a portion of media at 25-27°C to check for fungal growth or microorganism survived autoclaving. If no growth is observed, media is free from contamination and can be used or stored in refrigerator properly for further use.

8.   If growth is seen, it means it is not sterile. Therefore, it must be discarded and fresh medium should be prepared.

b. Preparation of nutrient agar medium:

1.   When the broth medium is supplemented with agar-agar, it is called agar medium.

2.   Generally, 1.5 to 2% agar-agar is added to the prepared broth and gently heated so as to dissolve agar-agar.

Uses:

Nutrient agar is a general purpose, nutrient medium which supports growth of a wide range of non-fastidious organisms. Nutrient agar is popular because it can grow a variety of bacteria and fungi.

Storage of Media:

1.   Media should always be stored in a cool moist place to prevent evaporation, preferably in the refrigerator. Prolonged storage of sterile media is not recommended.

2.   If media have been stored for a long time, they should be reheated in a boiling water bath for a few minutes, to drive off dissolved gases, and then cooled quickly in cold water without agitation prior to inoculation.

3. Agar tubes should be melted and allowed to solidify in order to secure a moist surface that is desired for most microorganisms. This can be done once. These precautions for both liquid and solid media are extremely important for the initiation of growth of microorganism.

The properties of agar which make it ideal in bacteriology are:

1. Agar-agar melts (dissolves) at 100°C.
2. Liquid agar solidifies at 42-44°C.
3. The percentage of agar to be added in the medium is 1.5-2%.
4. Semi-solid media contain 0.05-0.3% agar.

Precautions:

1. Over cooking of the media may not support the growth of the desired organism.
2. No media ingredient should be added in excess as excess ingredients may be growth inhibitory or toxic to microorganisms.

Nutrient broth medium

Petone-5g

Beef extract-3.0

Distilled water-1000mL

pH-7.0

Nutrient agar medium

Add 1.5 to 2% agar-agar to prepared nutrient broth and gently heated so as to dissolve agar-agar.

12

Aseptic Technique and Transfer of Microorganisms

Aseptic technique is the procedure followed to minimize or eliminate microbial contamination and maintain sterile conditions by any means. It is the most important and fundamental skill in the microbiology laboratory. This technique is used for performing all microbiological operations like inoculation of media, isolation of pure cultures, sub-culturing, transferring of cultures etc. There is no work done in the microbiology laboratory without following aseptic technique. Use of proper aseptic technique prevents contamination of cultures from foreign bacteria and fungi inherent in the environment.

General guidelines of aseptic technique:

1. Wash your hands with soap water both before and after lab work.
2. Pull back long hair or use a hair cover. Long hair is a potential source of contamination. Additionally, long hair could be a health hazard when working near an open flame.
3. Wear a lab coat and have your goggles on.
4. Rings, watches etc., should be removed from hands before carrying out aseptic technique.
5. Always disinfect the LAF bench before and after use with 70% ethanol.
6. First transfer all the requirements you need for the experiment by wiping the surface of LAF with 70% ethanol.
7. Work quickly and efficiently when carrying out aseptic technique.
8. When working, place test tubes in racks. Never lay down the tubes as they may leak.
9. Dump any microbial suspension in discard area only.

10. Flood the area of the spill with disinfectant and leave on for 10 minutes before using paper towel to soak up.

11. Label all the test tubes, Petri plates properly with date, the name of the organism and with experiment name using glass marker.

a. Bunsen burner:

It is a type of gas burner used in microbiology lab which provides blue coloured flame when adjusted. The burner is used to sterilize the inoculating needle, loop, mouth of the tubes; flasks etc. by passing over the flame to prevent the contamination of the air. All the microbial operations are done in the vicinity of Bunsen burner. The heat of the Bunsen burner also causes the air around the work to rise, reducing the chance of airborne contamination.

b. Sterilizing a inoculation loop:

The inoculating loop is sterilized by holding it at an angle in the flame of a Bunsen burner until the entire length of the wire becomes red hot from heat. By this, all the contaminants on the loop are incinerated. Now allow the loop to cool before picking up the inoculum as a hot loop may kill the inoculum. Never lay down the loop once it is sterilized as it may lead to contamination.

c. Flaming the mouth of the test tubes:

The mouth of the test tubes, flasks containing culture and fresh media tubes are passed through the flame of Bunsen burner. This creates a convection current which forces air out of the tube preventing airborne contaminants from entering the tube.

Aseptic Transfer of Microorganisms:

The procedure for aseptically transferring of microorganisms is as follows:

a.   Transfer of culture from broth to fresh broth

b.   Transfer of culture from broth to fresh slant

c.   Transfer of culture from broth to agar deep

d.   Transfer of culture from agar slant to a fresh broth

e.   Transfer of culture from agar plate to a fresh broth

Requirements:
  24 hour bacterial culture broth, agar tube, agar plate
  Sterile nutrient agar slants/broth/plates/flasks
  Inoculating loop
  Inoculation needle
  Glass marker
  Laminar air flow
  95% ethanol

a. Transfer of culture from broth to fresh broth:

Procedure:

1. Clean laminar air flow bench with 70% ethanol.
2. Wipe the outer surface of the materials required with 70% propanol and transfer to the left side of laminar air flow bench in a place where you reach them easily.
3. Hold both, the source culture tube and sterile broth tube in left hand. Be sure that all the tubes are labeled properly.
4. Hold the inoculating loop with the right hand, sterilize it on the flame of Bunsen burner at an angle so that wire of the loop turns red hot, now cool the wire and by holding the sterile inoculation loop in your right hand, remove cotton plugs of both the tubes by grasping them between the fingers.
5. Be sure to cool the inoculation loop before picking the inoculum from source culture tube.
6. Run the tops of both the tubes through the flame to take away the air contaminants from the tube entrance.
7. Shake the source culture tube and insert the inoculating loop to obtain a loopful of culture.
8. Introduce the loop containing inoculum quickly into the sterile tube so that the loop gets immersed into broth resulting in the transfer of culture from source to sterile broth in the tube.
9. Sterilize the inoculation loop to red hot on the burner again.
10. Pass the mouth of both the tubes through the flame again and replug with cotton plugs.
11. Incubate all the tubes at 37°C for 24-48 hours.

b. Transfer of culture from broth to fresh slant:

1. Hold the tubes in your left hand and follow the same aseptic techniques as described for broth transfer.

2. Shake the source culture tube and insert the inoculating loop to obtain a loopful of culture.

3. Inoculate the slant by streaking along the surface of the slant by moving the inoculation loop gently in a zig-zag fashion.

4. Label the tubes and incubate at 37°C for 24-48 hours and observe the growth.

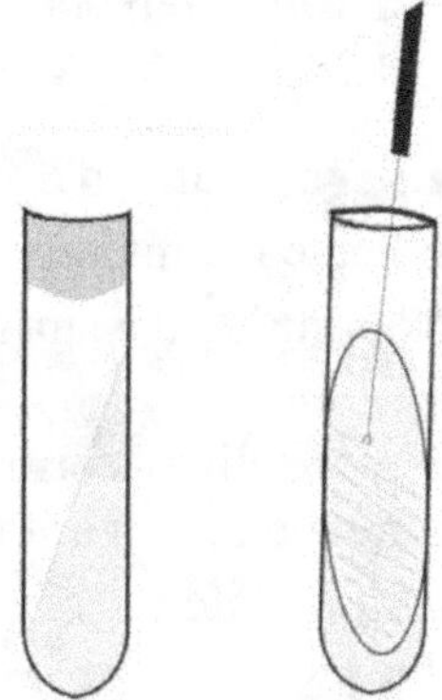

Figure showing slant inoculation by streaking

c. Transfer of culture from broth to agar stabs(deep):

1. Label the tubes properly with glass marker.

2. Hold the tubes in left hand as described earlier and sterilize the inoculating needle over the flame of Bunsen burner.

3. By following the aseptic procedure, dip the inoculating needle in to the tube containing culture broth.

4. Now stab the agar tube by thrusting the needle straight down into the agar center.

5. Plug the agar tube with cotton plug by following aseptic procedure.

6. Incubate the tubes at 37°C for 24-48 hours.

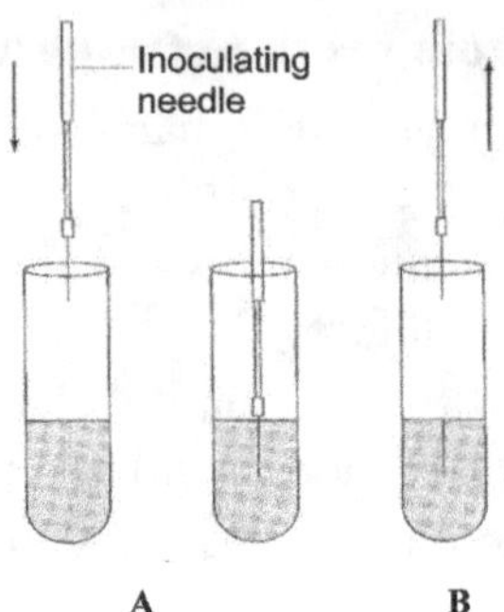

Figure showing stab inoculation

A. Stab inoculation by inoculation needle; B. Inoculated stab culture tube

d. Transfer of culture from agar slant to a fresh broth:

1. Label the tubes to indicate the microorganisms used.
2. Hold the tubes containing agar slant culture and sterile nutrient broth in left hand.
3. Follow the aseptic steps like sterilizing the inoculation loop, unplugging and flaming the mouth of the tubes as described earlier.
4. Insert the inoculating loop into the slant and obtain a small portion of the surface growth.
5. Immerse the inoculation loop containing the inoculum into the tube containing nutrient broth and shake gently to free the microorganisms adhere to it.
6. Flame the mouth of the tubes again and replace the cotton plugs into the respective tubes.
7. Flame the inoculating needle and put it down in a suitable place.
8. Incubate at 37°C for 24 hours and observe the growth.

e. Transfer of culture from agar plate to a fresh broth:

Procedure:

1. Select an agar plate with bacterial colonies. Mark the colony to be transferred with a marker on the underside of the Petri plate.
2. Sterilize the inoculating loop as described earlier and allow it to cool.
3. Open the lid of Petri plate slightly and pick up the selected colony with inoculation loop. Remove the cotton plug of the sterile broth tube carefully and pass the mouth of the tube on the flame.

4. Now inoculate the broth with inoculation loop containing culture so that the wire gets dipped in the broth. Shake the loop gently to free the microbes adhered to it.

5. Sterilize the inoculating loop and place in proper space.

6. Flame the neck of the tube and replace the plug and incubate at 37°C for 24 hrs.

Precautions:

1. Tubes, flasks and plates must be labeled properly with date and with name of the organism.

2. To prevent possible confusion, plates are marked on the underside while tubes and bottles must be labeled on the side.

3. Never lay down the cotton plugs as they may get contaminated.

4. Sterilize the inoculation loop and needle before and after use.

5. Allow the inoculation loop to cool down after passing through flame as hot loop will kill the microbes to be transferred.

6. Never place a contaminated loop on the table.

7. Work quickly and efficiently to minimize the time the culture is exposed to the environment.

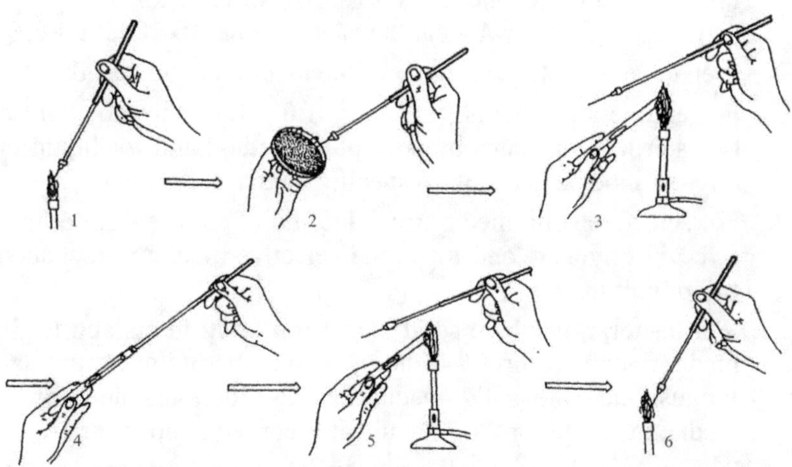

Figure showing culture transfer of plate to slant

1. Sterilizing inoculating loop; 2. Picking up colony to be transferred from plate;
3. Sterilizing the mouth of the slant; 4. Inoculating the culture to slants;
5. Flaming the mouth of the tube; 6. sterilizing the inoculating loop.

13

Growth Promotion Test of the Medium

Growth promotion test of microbiological culture media is to check whether the procured or prepared medium supports the growth of microbial cultures or not.

Requirements:

Saline (0.85% NaCl)

24 hours microbial cultures

Agar medium plates to be tested

Broth tubes to be tested

Procedure:

1. Prepare dilution of the microorganism specific for the medium to be tested in such a way that the bacteria give 10-100cfu/mL.

2. Prepare agar plates and broth of the medium to be tested.

3. For enumeration media, inoculate 1.0 mL of the inoculum on to two sterile agar plates by pour plate method and for liquid media directly inoculate 1.0mL to specific media.

4. For selective solid media streak loopful of culture from dilution of selected organism and for liquid selective medium inoculate loop full of culture.

5. For bacteria, incubate solid media for 24-72 hours and for liquid media, incubate for 18-48 hours at specified temperature and for fungus, incubate solid media for 72-120 hours and for liquid media, incubate for 24-72 hours at specified temperature.

6. Simultaneously maintain a positive control of the previously approved medium by using same quantity of inoculum used for test.

7. Similarly, maintain a negative control to check the testing conditions.

8. At the end of the incubation period observe the plates and count the number of bacterial colonies on both the plates and express the result in cfu by following formula.

$$\frac{P_1 + P_2}{2}$$

Where P_1 = plate 1

P_2 = plate 2

Calculate the microbial recovery using equation:

$$\% \text{ recovery} = \frac{\text{mean cfu observed} \times 100}{\text{inoculated cfu mL}}$$

If recovery is less than 70% media is not suitable for experiments.

Note: Solid medium should be compared with positive control and test media recovery should be not less than 70 %.

Note: For liquid media check the turbidity by comparing with positive control.

	Name of the media	Organism to be inoculated	Incubation period	Incubation temperature
1.	Nutrient agar	*Bacillus subtilis* *Candidaalbicans* *Staphylococcus aureus* *Pseudomonas aureus* *Aspergillus niger*	24-48 hours	30-35°C
2.	MacConkey agar	*E.coli*	24-48 hours	30-35°C
3.	Sabourauds Dextrose agar	*Candidaalbicans* *Aspergillus niger*	72-120 hours	20-25°C for fungi
4.	Soyabean casein Digest agar	*Bacillus subtiles* *Staphylococcus aureus* *C.albicans* *A-niger*	24-72 hours for bacteria and 72-120 hours for fungi	30-35°C for bacteria 20-25°C for fungi
5.	Eosin Methylene Blue agar	*E.coli*	24-48 hours	30-35°C

14

Preparation of Agar Slants, Stabs and Plates

Requirements:

Nutrient agar medium

Test tubes

Cotton plugs

Pipette

Water bath

Autoclave

Glass rod

Laminar air flow

Incubator

Procedure:

1. Place the test tubes in test tubes rack.

2. Prepare nutrient agar medium as described in media preparation section and boil it with stirring until the melted agar is distributed throughout the medium.

3. Transfer about 5mL of molten agar medium into each test tube using a pipette.

4. Now place the cotton plugs to the agar tubes.

5. Sterilize the agar tubes using autoclave at 121°C for 15 minutes at 15lbs pressure.

6. After sterilization, remove the tubes from autoclave and place in a slanting position to a solid support to get sufficient surface area and allow the medium to solidify.

7. Incubate the tubes at 37°C for 24-48 hours to check for any contamination of the slants.

8. When no contamination is found the slants can be used.

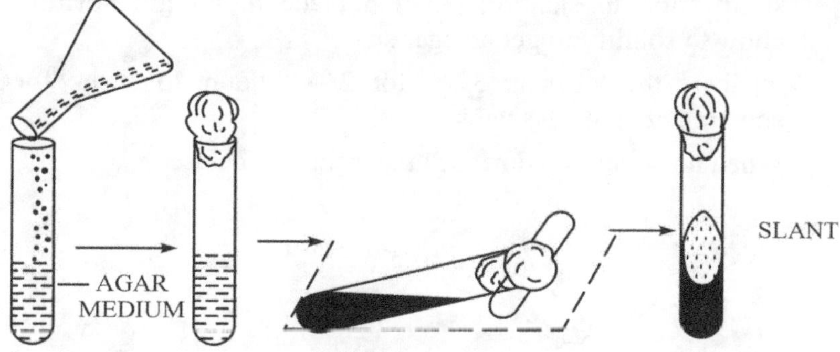

Preparation of agar slant

Precautions:

1. All work should be done by following the aseptic procedure.

2. Sterilization of agar medium should be done after adding into the tubes.

3. Place the agar tube in slanting position at an angle to give sufficient surface area.

4. Care should be taken to see that the medium does not touch the cotton plug while placing the tubes in slanting position.

Preparation of Agar Stabs

Requirements:

Nutrient agar medium

Test tubes

Cotton plugs

Pipette

Water bath

Autoclave

Glass rod

Laminar air flow

Incubator

Procedure:

1. For the preparation of agar stabs, follow the same procedure as described for agar slants but instead of placing the agar tubes after sterilization in slanting position place in upright position and allow to solidify to get an agar stab.

2. Incubate the tubes at 37°C for 24-48 hours to check for any contamination of the stabs.

3. When no contamination is found stabs can be used.

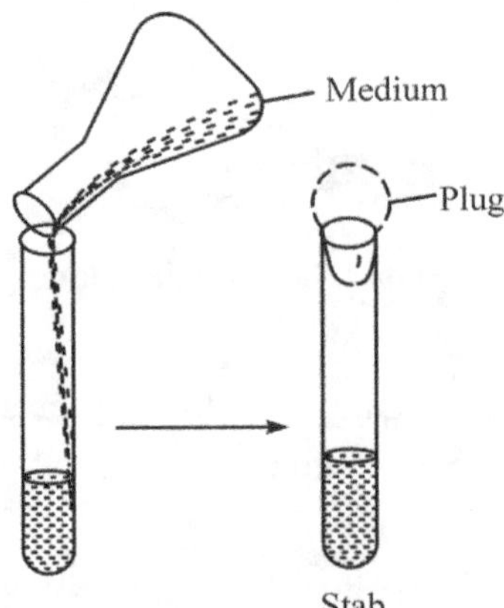

Preparation of agar stabs

Precautions:

1. All work should be done aseptically.

2. Sterilization of agar medium should be done after adding into the tubes.

3. Care should be taken that the medium does not touch the sides of the tubes while dispensing.

Preparation of Agar Plates

Requirements:

Nutrient agar medium

Sterile Petri plates

Test tubes (20mL capacity)

Cotton plugs

Pipette

Water bath

Autoclave

Glass rod

Laminar air flow

Incubator

Procedure:

1. Prepare nutrient agar medium as described in media preparation section and boil it with stirring until the melted agar is distributed throughout the medium.

2. Transfer about 15-20mL of molten agar medium into each test tube of 20mL capacity using a pipette.

3. Now place the cotton plugs to the agar tubes and sterilize using autoclave at 121°C for 15 minutes at 15lbs pressure.

4. After sterilization, remove the tubes from the autoclave and cool to 45°C and pour the medium quickly and carefully into the sterile Petri plates by raising the lid of the plate with left hand far enough to permit the mouth of the tube to enter without touching the sides, soon the tube is withdrawn and the lid is replaced and the plate is tilted to allow homogenous spreading of the medium and allow to solidify.

5. Incubate the agar plates at 37°C in an inverted position for 24-48 hours to check for any contamination.

6. When no contamination is found agar plates can be used.

Precautions:

1. All work should be done aseptically.

2. The plates should be placed in an inverted position in an incubator so that the moisture drops do not fall on the medium.

3. During pouring of the medium, care should be taken that the mouth of the tube does not touch any part of the Petri plate.

4. Do not pour hot medium into the plates.

5. Pour only 15-20 mL of the agar medium into Petri plates.

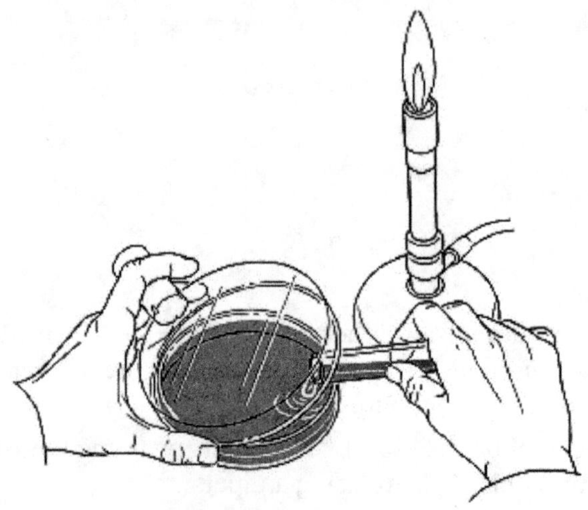

Preparation of agar plates

Nutrient agar medium

Peptone-5g

Beef extract-3.0

Agar-agar-15g

Distilled water-1000mL

pH-7.0

15

Preservation of Microbial Cultures

Microbial cultures are preserved in microbiological laboratories so that the cultures may be made available when required. Microbial culture preservation aims at maintaining a microbial strain alive, contamination free and without any mutation like the original culture. Different microorganisms can be preserved by different methods.

The technique of preservation of microbes is broadly classified in to two types:

1. Methods where organisms are in continuous metabolic active state.

2. Methods where organisms are in suspended metabolic state.

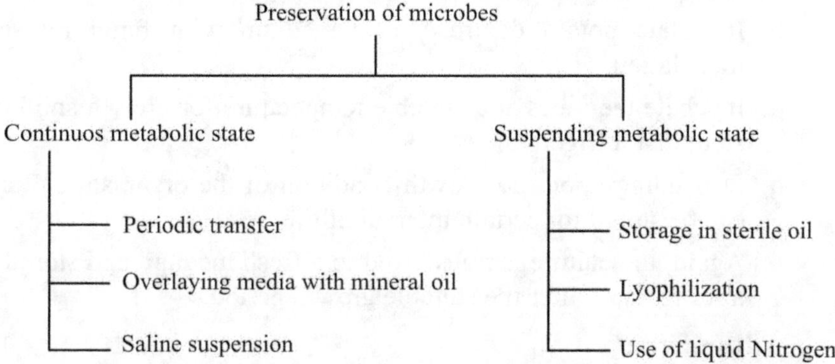

1. Methods where organisms are in continuous metabolic active state:

In this technique, organisms are preserved on appropriate medium by repeated sub-culturing. Here, sub-culturing is required due to depletion of nutrients or drying of the medium.

This technique includes following methods

a. Periodic transfer to fresh medium (sub-culturing):

Sub-culturing is the transfer of inoculum of the culture to a fresh medium.

Requirements:

Nutrient agar slants

Potato dextrose agar slants

Inoculation loop

Inoculation needle

Bunsen burner

Procedure:

1. Prepare nutrient agar and potato dextrose agar slants and allow them to solidify, check for sterility by incubating in an incubator.

2. Following aseptic technique, inoculate nutrient agar slants with bacterial culture by streaking on the slope of the agar medium.

3. Inoculate potato dextrose agar medium with fungi by spot inoculation.

4. Incubate the tubes at a suitable temperature for growth and later store in a refrigerator.

5. Depending upon the growth condition of the organism cultures can be stored for certain interval of time.

6. Again, the culture is transferred to a fresh medium and stored in a refrigerator after the suitable growth period.

Advantages:

1. Simple process. No need of any special apparatus

2. Easy to recover the culture

Disadvantages:

1. Chances of contamination are more

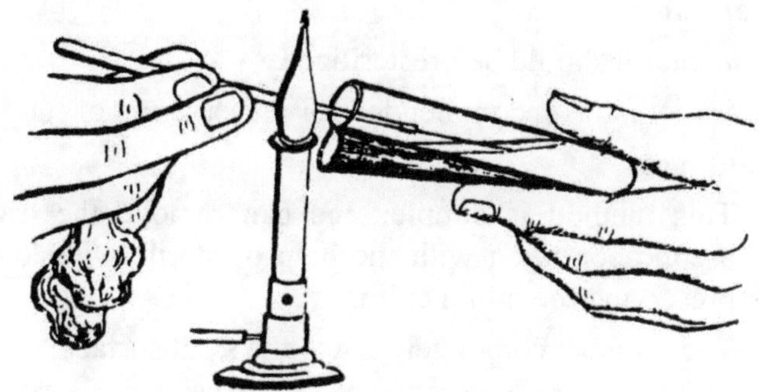

Method of subculturing

b. **Overlaying media with mineral oil:**

Requirements:

Nutrient agar slants

Potato dextrose agar slants

Inoculation loop

Inoculation needle

Bunsen burner

Pre sterilized Mineral oil or liquid paraffin

Procedure:

1. Prepare nutrient agar and potato dextrose agar slants and allow to solidify, checking for sterility by incubating in incubator at respective temperatures.

2. Following aseptic technique, inoculate nutrient agar slants with bacterial culture by streaking on slope of the agar medium.

3. Inoculate potato dextrose agar medium with fungi by spot inoculation.

4. Incubate the tubes at suitable temperature for growth.

5. When sufficient growth is seen they are covered with sterile mineral oil to a depth of 1 cm above the tip of the surface using aseptic conditions and store in refrigerator.

6. Revive the culture by picking a small bit of fungal culture and sub-culturing on a fresh slant, incubate at a suitable temperature.

7. When sufficient growth is seen the culture can be reused.

Precautions:

1. Mineral oil should be presterilized.

2. This method is recommended for preservation of fungal cultures

Advantages:

1. This method is simple; one can remove the organisms in aseptic condition with the help of sterile wire loop and still preserving the initial culture.

2. The oil must completely cover the slant surface.

3. The layer of mineral oil prevents dehydration of the medium.

4. The microorganisms remain in dormant state.

c. Saline suspension

Requirements:

24 hour bacterial slant culture

Inoculation loop

Bunsen burner

NaCl

Test tubes

Distilled water

Procedure:

1. Prepare saline solution by dissolving 0.85g of NaCl in 100 ml of distilled water and distribute 5.0 ml each into test tubes.

2. Sterilize using autoclave at 121°C for 15 minutes.

3. After sterilization cool the saline tubes to room temperature.

4. Inoculate a loopful of bacterial culture in to saline tube, shaken well and used.

Advantages:

1. Very useful for immediate use of bacterial culture.

2. Simple and inexpensive.

3. Saline provides proper osmotic pressure to organisms.

2. Methods where organisms are in suspended metabolic state:

a. Storage in sterile soil:

Requirements:

Sterile soil

Fungal cultures with spores

Agar slant of fungal cultures with spores

Sterile distilled water

Sterile soil

Sterile bottle

Procedure:

1. Grow the fungal culture on a suitable solid medium till it forms spores.
2. Suspend the spores in 1ml sterile water.
3. Transfer the culture suspension in to sterile soil in a bottle and allow the culture to grow for 10 days.
4. Later, store the bottle in a refrigerator for further use.
5. Revive the culture by dusting few soil particles on a suitable medium and incubating till it accomplishes optimum growth.

Note: This method is suitable especially for the fungi

b. Lyophilization or freeze drying:

This is the process of removing water from culture after it is frozen and then placed under vacuum. This process is widely used for long term preservation of bacteria, yeasts and fungi. In this process, water is removed by sublimation from the prefrozen culture. After drying, the powdered form of the culture is stored under vacuum in individual vials or ampoules. The suspending medium is very important factor for the cells to be lyophilized. Skimmed milk is commonly used. However, in place of skim milk, sucrose, glucose or serum is used in special cases.

Requirements:

Freezer (-20 and -80°C)

Lyophilizer

Skim milk broth (10g skim milk, in100ml H_2O sterilize)

Microbial cultures to be lyophilized, Pasteur pipette, glass ampoules

Procedure:

1. First, grow the microbial cultures in a Petri dish or agar slant containing suitable medium.

2. Overlay the culture with 4ml of 10% skim milk broth.

3. Make the suspension of the culture using Pasteur pipette.

4. Transfer the suspension quickly to sterilized vials by pipetting about 1.5 ml of the suspension and seal the mouth of the ampoule/vial with rubber cap.

5. Keep the ampoules in a -20°C freezer at first for 1-2 days and then in a -80 °C freezer for 24h.

6. Once the cultures are frozen, prepare the freeze-dryer by turning it on and allowing for the appropriate temperature and vacuum conditions to stabilize.

7. Place the vials into freeze drying cabinet of the lyophilizer and start the vacuum pump, allow the culture to dry out completely (lyophilize) which may take few hours (about 5 hours) to overnight depending on the volume of the sample.

8. Now again insert the ampoule into the ports of lyophilizer for secondary drying.

9. Finally, seal the ampoule/vials under vacuum on the dryer manifold.

10. Store the ampoules in the refrigerator for further use.

11. When needed, cultures can be revived by opening ampoule and adding 0.5ml of nutrient broth to make a suspension and transferring to a suitable medium and incubating for the growth of the culture.

Advantages:

1. Required minimum space for storage. Hundreds of lyophilized vials can be stored in a small area.

2. Vials can be sent conveniently to other laboratories by post.

c. Storage in liquid nitrogen:

This is an alternative method for long term preservation of microbial cultures apart from lyophilization. It is used especially in case of some of the microbial cultures which do not survive freeze drying. Further, some microbes do not tolerate the effect of repeated cooling and warming cycles such loss is reduced by the use of cryoprotectants such as glycerol, dimethyl sulfoxide (DMSO), and the adjustment of growth conditions, rate cooling and warming.

Procedure:

1. Grow the bacterial cells on their growth supportive agar medium in a Petri plate.

2. Overlay the cultures with 4ml of 5% of glycerol(v/v) or 5% DMSO on the growing culture plate.

3. Scrap the culture with the help of Pasteur pipette and make suspension of the culture.

4. Pour 0.5 ml of the cell suspension in to cryo-tube meant for storage.

5. Transfer and store the culture in liquid nitrogen after proper labeling.

6. Culture can be revived by keeping it at room temperature for 2-3 hours and thereafter transfer onto suitable media under aseptic conditions.

7. Incubate the media containing plates at appropriate temperature for 24 hours or till growth appears.

Advantages:

1. Cultures can be stored for 10 to 30 years without undergoing any change in their characteristics.

Disadvantages:

1. This method is expensive.

16

Streak Plate Method

In nature, bacteria exist generally in mixed form and to study cultural, morphological and physiological characters of an individual bacterial species, it is important to get them separated from the mixed population of cells and get them in pure form.

The simple methods for isolation of pure culture include:

1. Streak plate method
2. Spread plate method
3. Pour plate method

1. Streak plate method for isolation of pure culture from mixed culture:

In streak plate technique individual colonies are isolated on the surface of an agar medium using an inoculating loop. Here, a loopful of culture is spread over the surface of solid agar medium so that the culture gets diluted while streaking over the agar medium to give well separated surface colonies. The idea is to obtain isolated pure colonies after incubation of the plate.

Requirements:

Mixed culture of bacteria

Wire loop

Nutrient agar medium

Sterile Petri plates

Laminar air flow/ Bunsen burner

Procedure:

1. Transfer all the requirements to a sterile environment such as laminar air flow preferably to left hand side.

2. Prepare nutrient agar plates as described earlier so that the medium is uniformly distributed.

3. Label the bottom of the Petri plate with date and other details.

4. Sterilize the inoculation loop over the flame of Bunsen burner until it turns red hot. Allow it to cool for few seconds, and aseptically transfer a loopful of the mixed culture to the edge of the agar plate.

5. Regardless of the type of streaking viz. radiant, T-streak, quadrant, continuously drag the loop gently to spread out the sample in the direction as shown in the figure without digging the agar. The loop is sterilized between different sets of streaks.

6. Incubate the plates at 37°C for 24 hours. Examine the growth of the colonies carefully.

7. Confluent growth is seen at the primary site of inoculum and well separated colonies appear on the final series of streaks.

8. All the separated colonies should have the same general appearance, if there is more than one type of colony, each type should be streaked again on a separate plate to obtain a pure culture.

Precautions:

1. Add 2% agar when preparing plates for streaking.

2. Do not dig the agar while streaking.

3. The inoculation loop is sterilized between different sets of streaks.

4. Label the Petri plate on the bottom rather than on the lid.

5. The lid of the agar plate has to be opened sufficient enough to streak the plate with the loop.

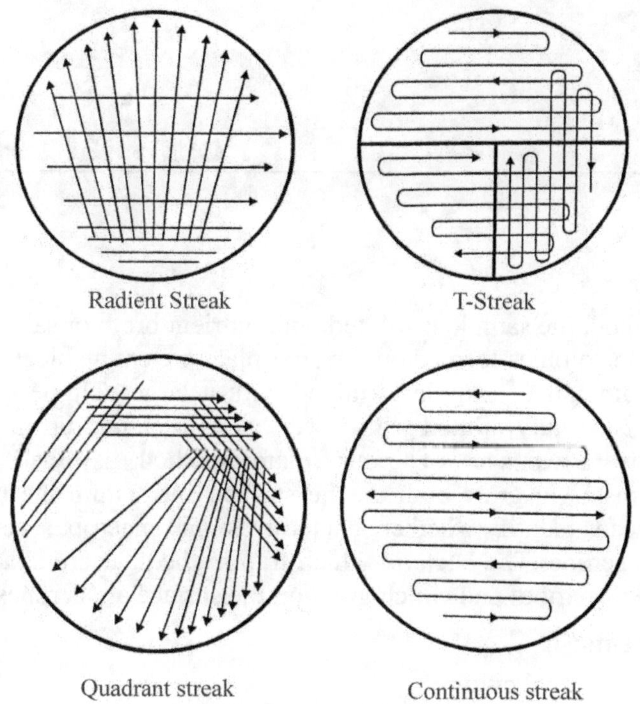

Various methods of streaking

17

Pour Plate Method

In this method, the sample is diluted with nutrient broth or saline in such a way that the colonies formed on the agar plate are countable. Generally, a measured amount of sample is mixed with a large volume of saline or broth and is serially diluted with fewer bacteria ending up in successive tubes. The advantage of pour plate method is that it allows microorganisms to grow both on the surface and within the medium so that, we can identify whether bacteria is an anaerobe, aerobe or a facultative aerobe. The bacteria which trap in the agar are anaerobes and facultative anaerobes and which grow on the surface are aerobes.

Requirements:

Mixed microbial culture

Physiological saline (0.85% NaCl)

Nutrient agar medium

Petriplates

Inoculation loop

Glass marker

Test tubes

Laminar air flow

Procedure:

1. Transfer all the sterilized materials into laminar air flow bench and mark the glassware properly.

2. Take 9.0 mL saline in 5 test tubes and inoculate the first tube with 1.0 mL mixed culture to be tested and after thorough mixing, the sample is serially diluted in saline. From the first tube (10^{-1}) 1mL is transferred to second test (10^{-2}) tubes and 1mL from the second

test tube is transferred to third test tube (10^{-3}) and the process is continued till 10^{-4}, 10^{-5} dilutions are achieved.

3. From the last three dilutions 1mL is poured into the center of sterile empty Petri plate using a sterile pipette. Meanwhile, the prepared nutrient agar (approx 15mL) cooled to 45°C is poured into the Petri plate containing the sample and the plate is rotated gently for uniform mixing of the sample in the agar medium.

4. After solidification of the agar, the plate is inverted and incubated at 37°C for 24-48 hours.

5. After the incubation period, well developed isolated bacterial colonies will be seen in last two dilutions.

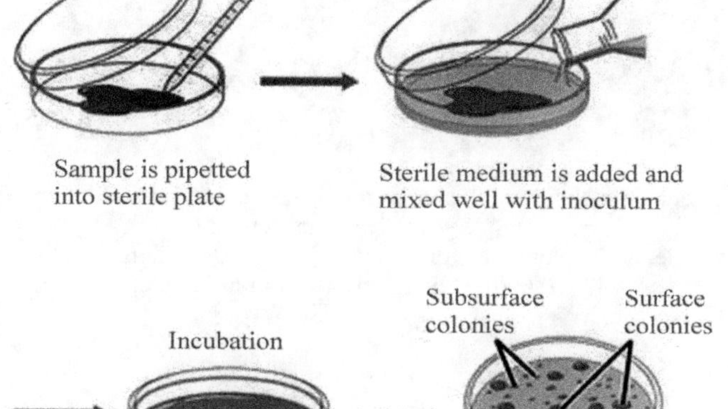

Pour plate method

Note:

The pour plate method apart from isolating pure cultures from mixed cultures, it is also used for determining the number of viable bacterial cells present in a sample.

The number of viable cells can be calculated according to the formula.

Number of bacteria per mL = Number of colonies on plate × dilution factor

For example: if 20 colonies are on 10^{-4} plate, then count is $20 \times 10,000 = 20000$ bacteria/mL

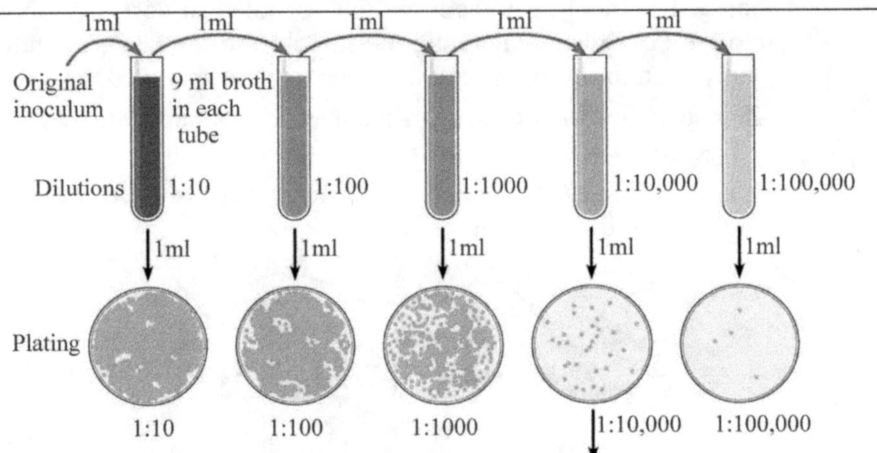

Calculation: Number of colonies on plate × reciprocal of dilution of sample = number of bacteria/ml

(For example, if 32 colonies are on a plate of 1/10,000 dilution, then the count is 32×10,000 = 320,000 bacteria/ml in sample.)

18

Spread Plate Technique

This is another dilution technique of isolation of pure culture from a mixed culture. In this technique, the number of bacteria per unit volume is reduced by serial dilution and a small amount of inoculum is spread over the solid agar medium in a Petri plate with an L-shaped sterile glass rod. A spread plate will have a countable number of bacterial colonies evenly distributed on the plate.

Requirements:

Mixed bacterial culture

Glass spreader (L-Shaped glass rod)

% propanol or 95% ethanol

Beaker

Saline or nutrient broth tubes

Pipettes

Procedure:

1. Prepare serial dilutions of the broth culture as described earlier. Be sure to mix the nutrient broth tubes/saline tubes before each serial transfer. Aseptically transfer 0.1 mL of the final three dilutions (10^{-5}, 10^{-6}, and 10^{-7}) to each of three nutrient agar plates.

2. Position the beaker of alcohol containing the glass spreader away from the flame. Remove the spreader and very carefully pass it over the flame just once. This will ignite the excess alcohol on the spreader and effectively sterilize it.

3. Remove the lid of the inoculated Petri plate and touch the sterile spreader to agar surface and move it back and forth while turning the plate. Repeat the process while spinning the plate till the inoculum is totally spread over the agar surface.

4. Replace the lid of the Petri plate and immerse the spreader in propanol and pass over the flame to sterilize.

5. Incubate the inoculated plates in an inverted position at 37°C for 24 hours.

Observation and Results: Well developed isolated colonies will be observed.

Precautions:

1. Always take last three dilution plates as first plates will be crowded with bacterial colonies.

2. Do not pipette out bacterial culture by mouth.

3. Sterilize glass spreader after spreading.

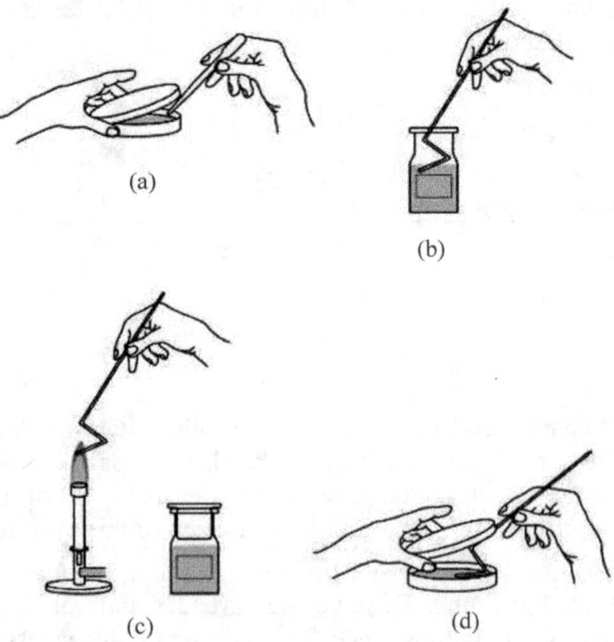

Figure showing the steps of spread plate technique

STAINING TECHNIQUES OF MICROORGANISMS

19

Preparation of a Bacterial Smear

A bacterial smear is a thin layer of bacteria placed on a glass slide for staining. The main goal of smear preparation is to place an appropriate concentration of bacterial cells on a slide and then cement them there so that they do not wash off during the subsequent staining procedure. The success of bacterial staining depends on the preparation of good smear. The smear can be prepared from liquid media or solid media.

a. From liquid culture

Requirements:

24 hours bacterial culture

Inoculating loop

Glass slide

Bunsen burner

Procedure:

1. Take a clean grease free glass slide, flame it over the burner, label it on one side and place it aside on LAF.

2. Take the liquid bacteria culture and shake the tube properly for uniform mixing of the culture.

3. By following aseptic technique, transfer a loop full of the culture over the clean glass slide and prepare a smear by spreading it in an anticlockwise direction.

4. Now allow the smear to air dry and later gently heat the slide by passing over the flame 2 to 3 times for fixing the smear on the slide.

From Liquid Medium

From Solid Medium

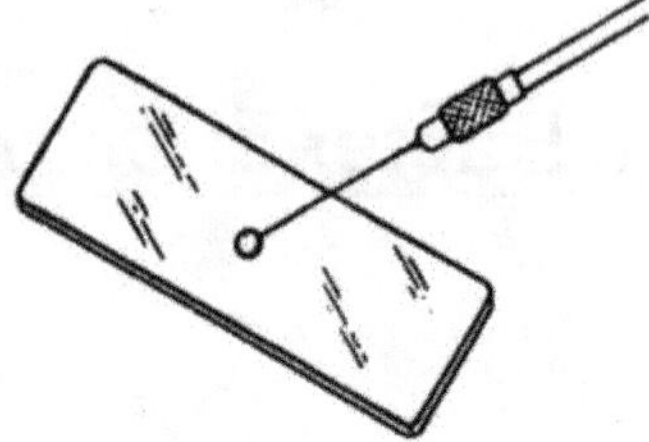

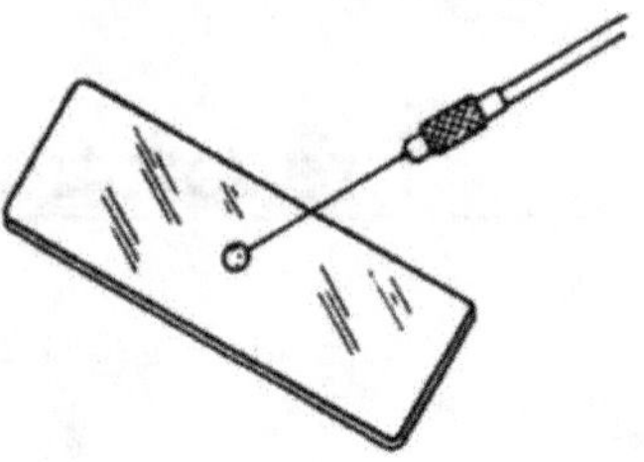

(a) Place a loopful of the cell suspension on a clean grease free slide

(a) Take one drop of water on the loop and place it on the center of the slide

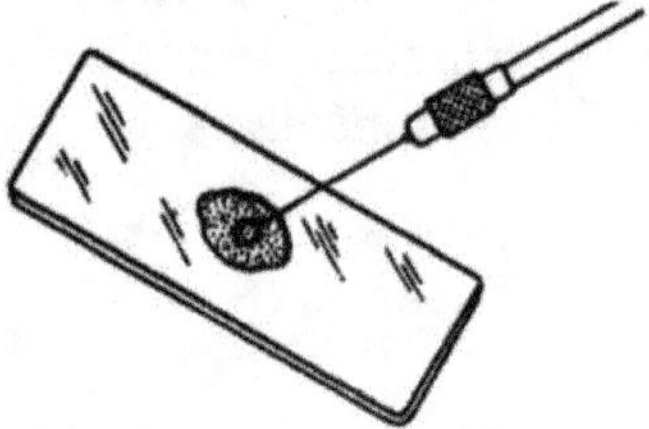

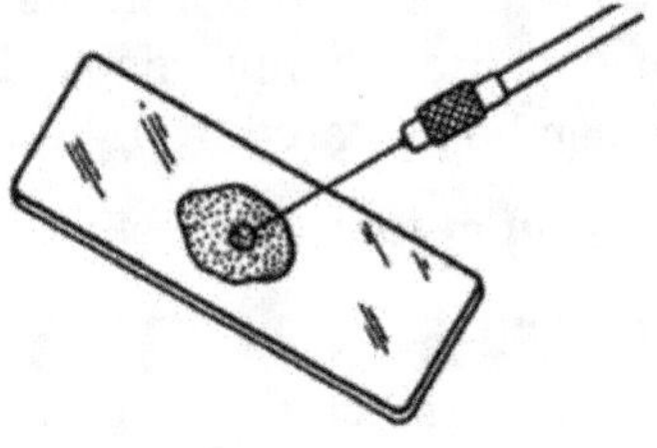

(b) With a circular movement of the loop spread the suspension into a thin area approximately the size of a dime

(b) Transfer a small amount of the bacterial inoculum from the slant culture into the drop of water. Spread both into a thin area approximately the size of a nickel.

Flxation

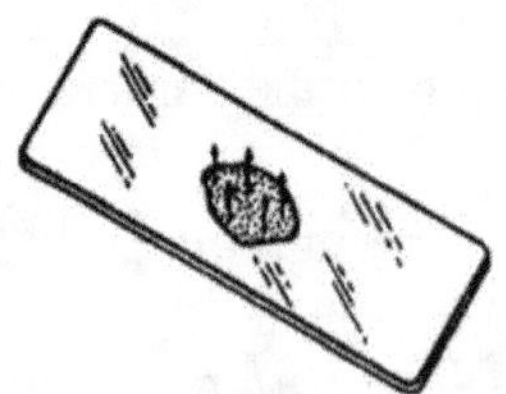

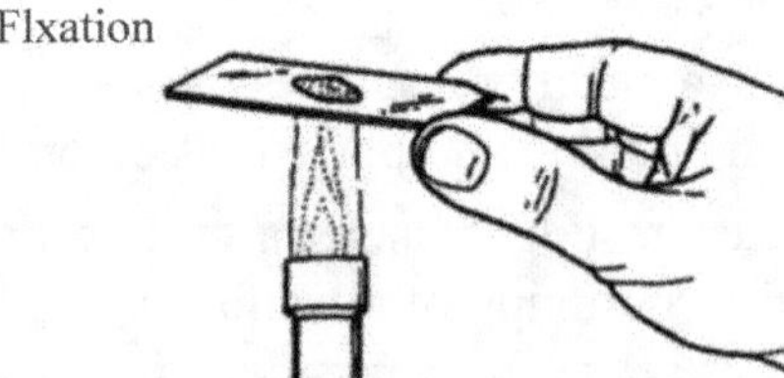

(c) Allow the smear to air dry

(c) While holding the slide at one end, quickly pass smear over the flame of the Bunsen burner two to three times.

Bacterial smear preparation

b. From solid culture
1.   Prepare the slide as describes above.
2.   Place a drop of water over the clean glass slide and transfer a small portion of the bacterial culture from agar slant following aseptic technique.
3.   Now prepare the smear as described and allow it to air dry.
4.   Gently heat the slide by passing over the flame 2 to 3 times for fixing the smear on the slide.

Precautions:
1.   For best visibility of bacteria, prepare smear by picking up bacteria from solid medium.
2.   Don't forget to heat fix the smear.

Heat fixing:
1.   Heat fixing kills bacteria that may still be alive.
2.   It also facilitates stain penetration.
3.   Heat fixing fixes cells to the slide so that they do not wash off while staining.

20

Staining

Most bacteria are colourless and transparent and have a refractive index similar to that of the aqueous fluids in which they are suspended. Owing to the small size of bacteria their structural details cannot be seen with the ordinary light microscope unless they are stained.

A stain is a dye consisting of a coloured ion (a chromophore) and a counter ion to balance the charge. Attachment of the chromophore part of the dye-complex to a cellular component represents the staining reaction. There are two types of dyes: cationic (basic) and anionic (acidic). Cationic dyes have a positively charged chromophore and high affinity for negatively charged cellular components. Since bacteria carry a net negative charge at pH 7, such dyes can be used to stain the cells directly. Some examples of cationic dyes are crystal violet, safranin, methylene blue and basic fuchsin. The other type of dyes, the anionic dye, has a negatively charged chromophore. The surface of bacteria at pH 7 repels such dyes and thus only the background is stained. After staining, cells would be seen as clear and bright bodies against a dark background. Such staining procedure is called negative staining. Nigrosin and eosin belong to this group of dyes.

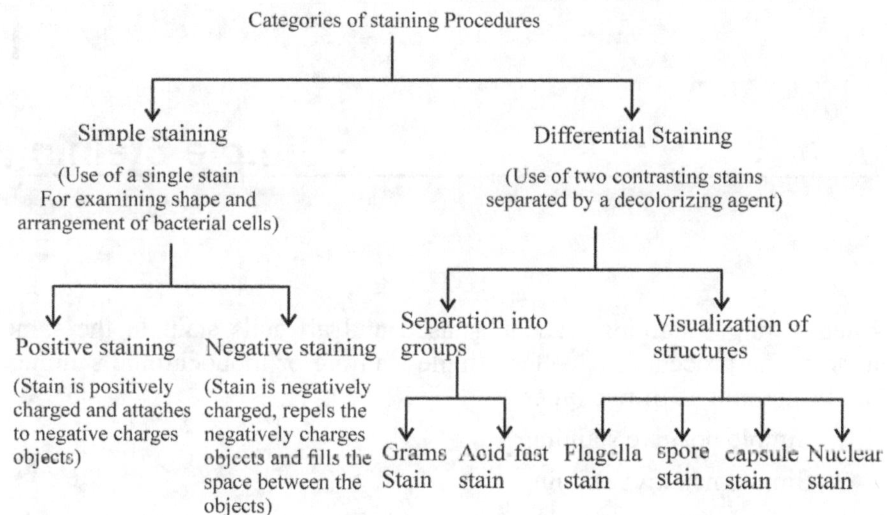
Categories of staining Procedures
Simple staining
(Use of a single stain
For examining shape and
arrangement of bacterial cells)
Differential Staining
(Use of two contrasting stains
separated by a decolorizing agent)
Positive staining
(Stain is positively
charged and attaches
to negative charges
objects)
Negative staining
(Stain is negatively
charged, repels the
negatively charges
objects and fills the
space between the
objects)
Separation into
groups
Visualization of
structures
Grams
Stain
Acid fast
stain
Flagella
stain
spore
stain
capsule
stain
Nuclear
stain

21

Simple Staining

When a single staining-reagent is used and all cells stain in the same manner, the procedure is called simple staining or monochrome staining. Simple staining is of two types.

1. Simple positive staining

2. Simple negative staining

In simple positive staining, staining is performed with basic dyes such as crystal violet, saffranin or methylene blue which have positively charged chromophore and are attracted to negatively charged bacterial cells.

In simple negative staining, staining is done using acidic, negatively charged (acidic) dyes such as nigrosin or Congo red which are repelled by the negatively charged bacteria and gather around the cells, leaving the cells clear and unstained.

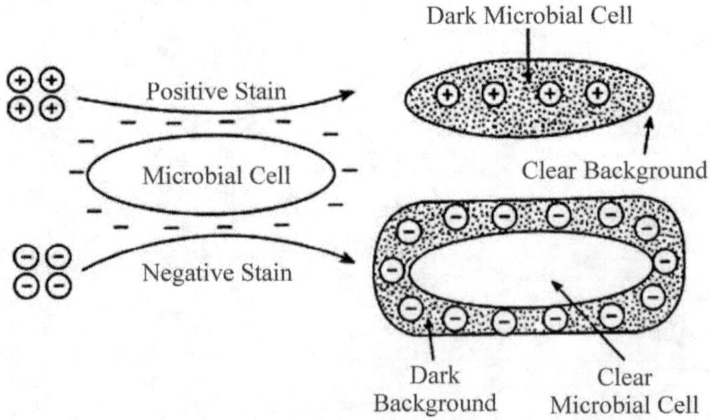

Simple positive and negative staining of bacterial cells

Simple Positive Staining

Materials required:

Bacterial culture of *Bacillus subtilis*

Inoculation loop

Glass slide

Bunsen burner

Staining tray

crystal violet or saffranin or methylene blue

Microscope

Immersion oil

Procedure:

1. Prepare the bacterial smear on a clean grease free glass slide and allow it to air dry.

2. Heat-fix the specimen on the glass slide, unless the specimen is heat-fixed, the bacterial smear will wash away during the staining procedure.

3. Flood the slide with crystal violet or saffranin or methylene blue and wait for 2 min.

4. Wash the smear with water to remove the excess stain.

5. Blot dry the slide and observe under 40 X objective lens of a microscope.

6. Later, add immersion oil and examine under 100X objective lens.

Observation and Results: Rod shaped bacteria are observed in violet or red or blue colour depending upon the stain used against colourless background.

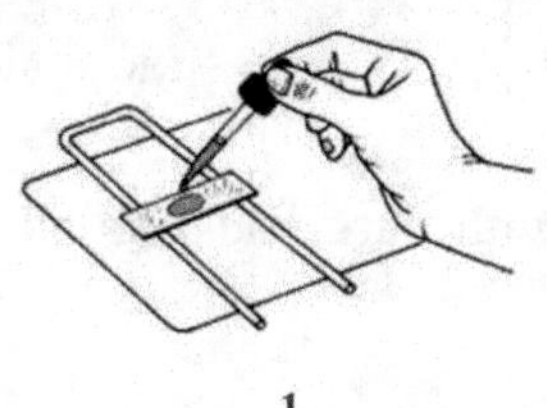

1

A bacterial smear is stained with methylene blue for one minute

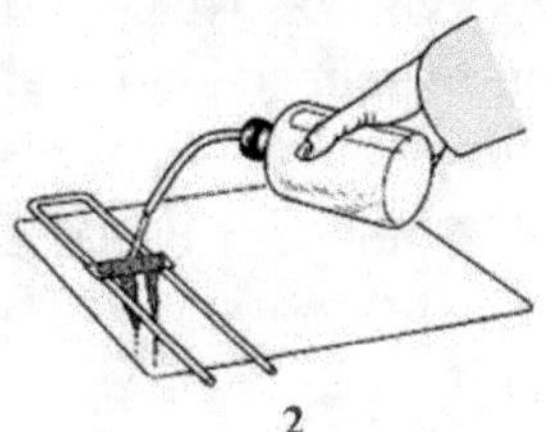

2

Stain is briefly washed off slide with water

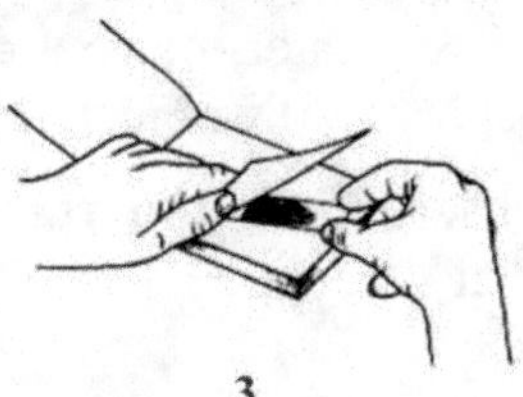

3

Water drops are carefully blotted off slide with bibulous paper

22

Negative Staining

Materials required:
- Bacterial culture
- Nigrosin or congo red
- Inoculating loop
- Glass slides
- Staining tray
- Microscope
- Bunsen burner

Procedure:
1. Place a small drop of nigrosin on one end of a clean glass slide.
2. Apply a small amount of the culture with an inoculating loop and disperse it in the drop of nigrosin.
3. Using the edge of another clean glass slide spread the drop of stain containing the bacteria across the slide by maintaining a small acute angle between the slides producing a broad, even, thin smear.
4. Allow the smear to air dry.
5. Observe under 40X objective lens of the microscope.
6. Later, place a drop of immersion oil and observe the slide under 100X objective lens.

Observation and results: Colourless bacteria with dark background is seen

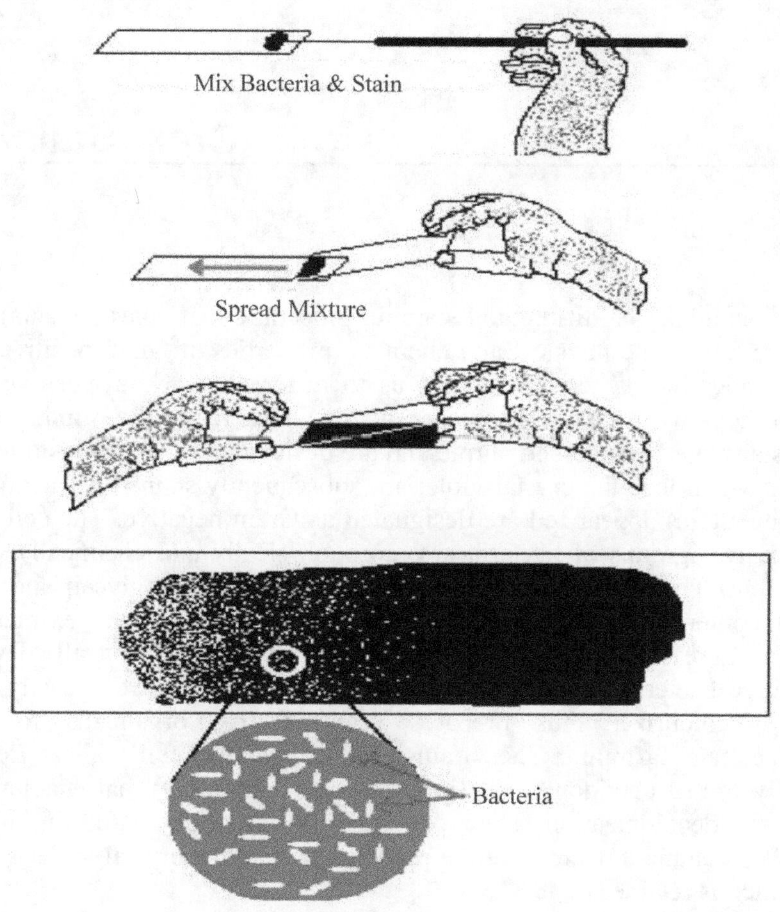

Negative staining

23

Gram Staining

Gram staining is a differential staining procedure that takes advantage of differences in the physical and chemical properties of Gram positive and Gram-negative bacteria. It allows us to differentiate Gram-positive and Gram-negative bacteria. Those organisms which retain the primary stain (crystal violet) are stained purple and are designated as Gram-positive and those which lose the crystal violet are subsequently stained by a safranin (counterstain) appear red are designated as Gram-negative. The cell wall of the two groups of bacteria are morphologically and chemically quite different. The gram negative cell wall has less peptidoglycan and high lipid content. During the decolonization step, alcohol may extract the lipids, increasing the porosity or permeability of the cell wall of gram negative bacteria. Thus, the crystal violet-iodine complex is easily lost. The decolourizer thus prepares gram-negative organisms for the counterstain saffranin. The Gram-positive bacterial cell wall is rich in tightly linked peptidoglycans (protein-sugar complexes) that enable cells to resist decolonization. Their cell walls become dehydrated during the alcohol treatment decreasing the porosity, so that the crystal violet-iodine complex is retained.

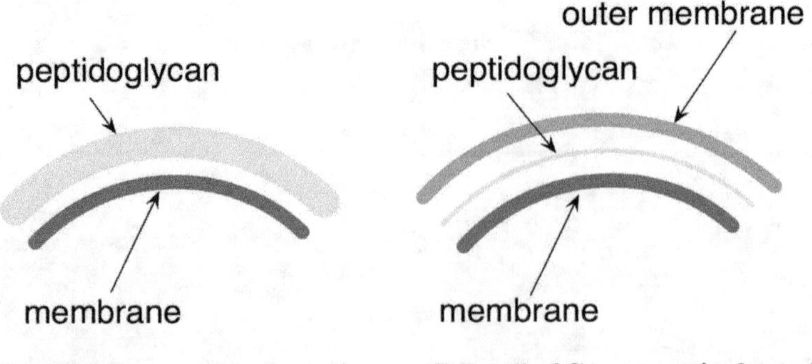

Cell wall of Gram positive bacteria   **Cell wall of Gram negative bacteria**

Materials Required:

24-hours broth cultures of *Bacillus subtilis, Escherichia coli*

Glass Slides

Inoculation loop

Staining tray

Bunsen burner

Gram's staining kit:
  a. Crystal Violet
  b. Grams Iodine
  c. Ethyl alcohol 95%
  d. Safranin

Immersion oil

Microscope

Procedures:

1. Prepare bacterial smear of each bacterial culture separately on a clean grease glass slide with the help of inoculation loop.

2. Air dry the smear and heat fix by passing over Bunsen burner flame.

3. Flood the slides with primary stain crystal violet and allow to stand for two minutes.

4. Wash off the stain with water and air dry.

5. Flood the smear with Gram's iodine (a mordant) and leave for one minute and again wash with water and air dry.

6. Decolourize the slide with alcohol (95%) for 10-20 seconds by keeping the slide in slanting position.

7. Wash with water and air dry it.

8. Counter stain the slide with safranin for one minute and wash with water and air dry.

9. Examine the preparation of both the slides first under 40X objective lens and later under the oil immersion (100X) objective lens of the microscope.

Observation and results:

a. The bacteria which appear purple in colour are Gram positive.

b. The bacteria which appear pink are Gram negative.

Precautions:

1. Decolonization is the most critical step. Be careful not to over decolorize, as many Gram-positive organisms may lose the violet stain easily and thus appear to be gram negative after they are counter stained with safranin.

2. On the underside of each slide, make a code mark so that slides can be identified.

3. Do not touch the slides to avoid transfer of bacteria from one slide to other.

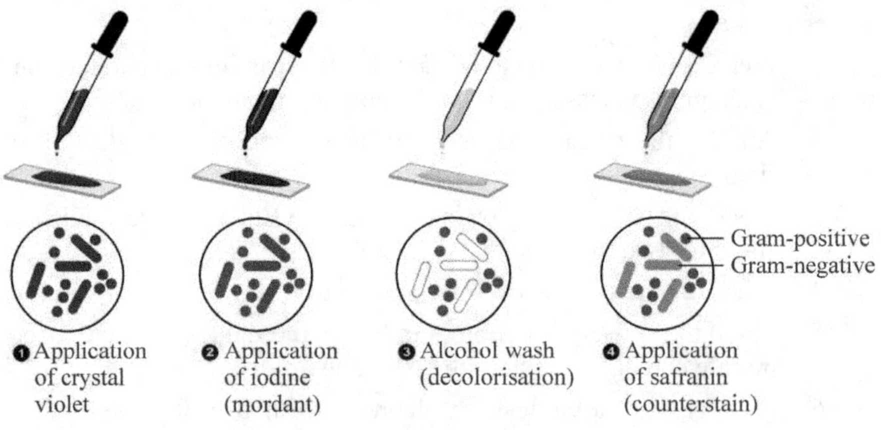

Gram staining procedure

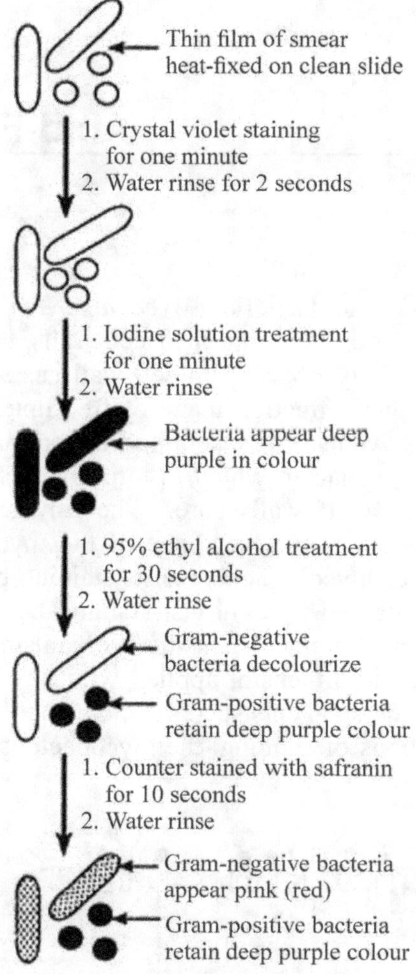

Mechanism of Grams staining

24

Acid-Fast Staining

Members of the certain bacteria (*Mycobacterium* spp.) contain large amounts of lipid substances within their cell walls, hence their cells have limited permeability. Mycobacterium cell wall has soluble and insoluble fractions. Where soluble fraction made of free lipids gets washed away when treated with solvents. The insoluble fraction made of peptidoglycan is attached to arabinogalactan which in turn is attached to mycolic acids (lipids) termed as cell wall core. The mycolyl arabinogalactan-peptidoglycan complex is the backbone of the mycobacterial cell wall. This large amount of mycolic acids resists staining by ordinary methods. They can only be stained by acid-fast staining by applying heat which helps in penetration of stain. When these organisms are stained with a basic dye, such as carbolfuchsin, applied with heat it cannot be readily removed even with harsh agents such as acid alcohol decolourizing agent. Under these conditions of staining, the mycobacteria are said to be acid-fast.

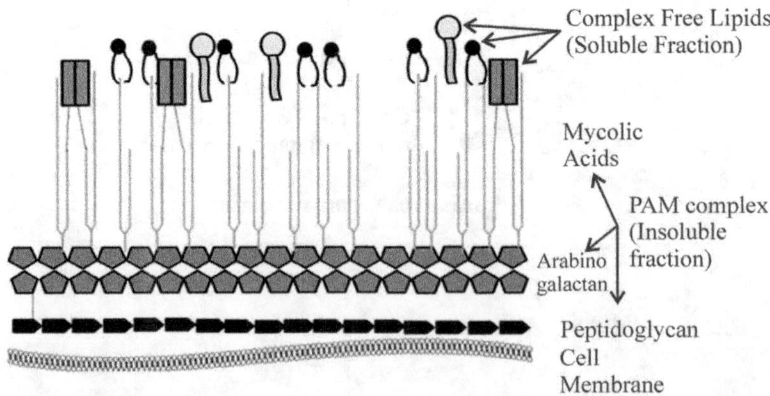

Representative diagram of the cell wall of Mycobacterium tuberculosis

The original technique for applying carbolfuchsin with heat is called the *Ziehl-Neelsen stain,* named after the two bacteriologists who developed it.

Requirements:

24-hour culture of *Bacillus subtilis*

Sputum sample of Tuberculosis patient

Carbol fuchsin stain (Primary stain)

*Acid alcohol Decolourizing solvent)

*(Ethanol 95%+ ConcHCl 3mLor 20%H_2SO4)

Methylene blue stain

Glass slides

Glass marker

Slide rack

Laminar air flow

Microscope

Immersion oil

Procedures

1. Prepare smears of both sputum sample and *B. subtilis,* air dry and heat-fixed by passing over the flame.

2. Place the slides on a slide rack on a metal staining tray.

3. Flood the slides with primary stain carbolfuchsin and allow standing for five minutes.

4. Heat the preparation gently by passing the Bunsen burner under the slide or steam over boiling water. Continue heating until steaming is observed.

5. Maintain steaming for five minutes. Add more dye as needed to prevent drying out of the smear.

6. Allow slides to cool, then rinse gently in running water.

7. Decolourize the slides with acid alcohol for 20 seconds and immediately wash with water using wash bottle and air dry.

8. Then counterstain the smear with methylene blue for 30 seconds to 1minute.

9. Wash gently using running water or with wash bottle, blot dry and observe under oil immersion (100X) objective lens.

Observation and results:

a. The bacterium *Mycobacterium tuberculosis* is positive for carbolfuchsin stain and appears red.

b. The other bacterium *Bacillus subtilis* is negative for this stain and take the counter stain methylene blue and appear blue.

Precautions:

1. Mark both the slides properly with glass marker to avoid confusion.

2. Take great care while heating carbolfuchsin to reduce the fire risk.

3. Do not touch the slides to avoid transfer of material.

Acid fast staining can also be applied to:

1. All *mycobacterium* are acid fast. Do not provide species identification.

2. Members of the Actinomycetes of genus *Nocardia* are partially acid fast.

3. Oocysts of coccidian parasite such as *Cryptosporidium* and *Isospora* are also acid fast.

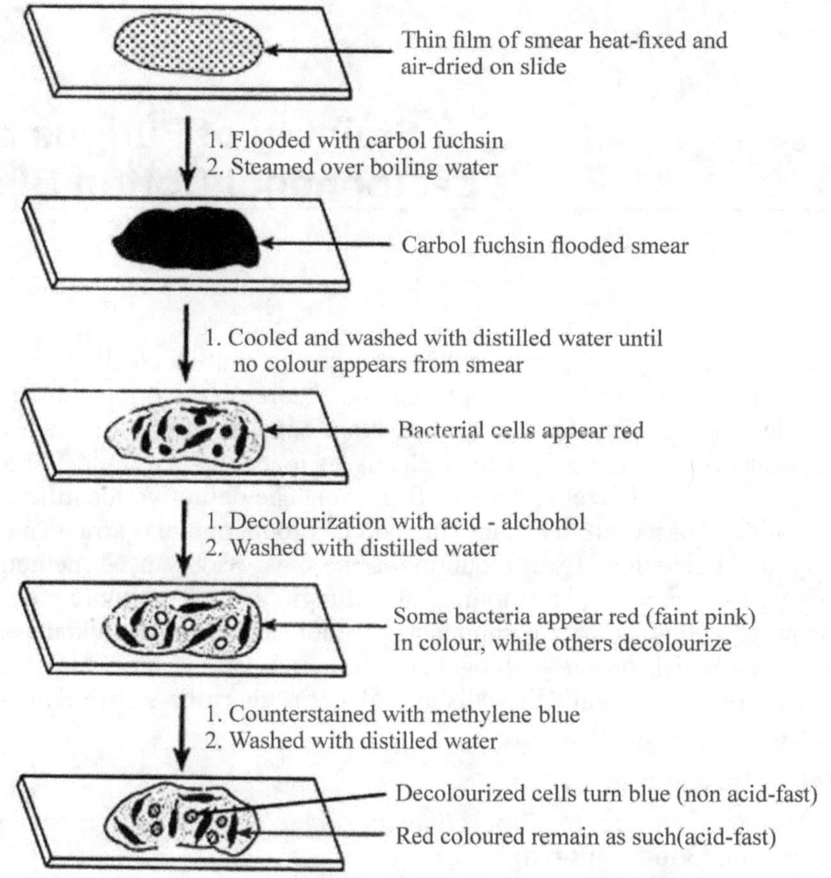

Acid-fast staining

25

Staining of Fungus by Lactophenol Cotton Blue

Fungi are eukaryotic single celled (yeast) or multinucleate (moulds) organisms which live by decomposing and absorbing the organic material in which they grow. The cell wall of fungi consists of chitin which is a polysaccharide composed of long chains of n-acetylglucasamine. It also contains other polysaccharides like B-glucan. The definitive identification of moulds is based on the shape, method of production and arrangements of spores. Lactophenol wet mounting is the most widely used method of staining and microscopic examination of fungi which is a simple process. The preparation has three components: phenol, serves as fungicidal agent, lactic acid which preserves fungal structure and cotton blue which stains the chitin in the fungal cell walls and glycerin gives the semi permanent preparation of the slide.

Materials required:

A young culture of *Aspergillus* or *Penicillium* growing on solid medium (3 to 5 days old).

Lactophenol cotton blue stain

Needles

Glass slides

Cover slips

Microscope

Procedure:

1. Place a drop of lactophenol cotton blue on a clean grease free slide.

2. With the help of sterile needle, aseptically remove a fragment of fungal colony and transfer into the lactophenol cotton blue on the slide and tease out the hyphae with the help of mounted needles.

3. Cover the preparation with a cover slide, taking care to avoid trapping of air bubbles in the lacto-phenol blue.

4. Examine the slide using the low (10X) and high power (40X) objectives.

5. Permanent slides can be made by using Dibutylphthalate polystyrenexylene (DPX) as sealing material.

Observation and results:

A lightly stained cytoplasm against unstained clear cell walls of hyphae, conidiophores, phialides and conidia of *Aspergillus* against light blue background can be seen.

Precautions:

1. Store lactophenol cotton blue at room temperature, avoid contact with eyes or skin.

2. Needles are to be sterilized before placing on LAF bench.

BIOCHEMICAL TESTS FOR IDENTIFICATION OF BACTERIA

26

IMViC Tests

IMViC Tests

IMViC is a series of tests used to study the physiological characteristics of bacteria from the family Enterobacteriaceae, especially *Escherichia* and *Enterobacter*. They are designed to differenciate Gram-negative intestinal bacilli of family Enterobacteriace which contains a large number of genera that are biochemically and genetically related to one another. IMViC tests consist of four different tests each of the letters in "IMViC" stands for one of these tests. "I" is for indole; "M" is for methyl red; "V" is for Voges-Proskauer, and "C" is for citrate, lowercase "i" is added for the ease of pronunciation.

IMViC Test results of Some Genera of Enterobacteriaceae:

1. IMViC tests of *Escherichia coli*
    1. Indole test: Positive
    2. Methyl-Red test: Positive
    3. Voges-Proskauer test: Negative
    4. Citrate test: Negative
2. IMViC tests of *Enterobacter aerogenes*
    1. Indole test: Negative
    2. Methyl-Red test: Negative
    3. Voges-Proskauer test: Positive
    4. Citrate test: Positive
3. IMViC tests of *Proteus vulgaris*
    1. Indole test: Positive
    2. Methyl-Red test: Positive
    3. Voges-Proskauer test: Negative
    4. Citrate test: Negative

4. IMViC tests of *Citrobacter freundii*
   1. Indole: Negative
   2. Methyl-Red: Positive
   3. Voges-Proskauer test: Negative
   4. Citrate test: Positive

27

Indole Test

Indole test is used to determine the ability of an organism to split tryptophan, an essential amino acid by using enzyme tryptophanase resulting in the formation of a compound called indole. The formation of Indole can be detected by addition of Kovac's or Ehrlich's reagent. Indole reacts with 4 (p)-dimethylamino benzaldehyde present in Kovac's reagent to give a red colour which concentrates as a ring at the top of the medium.

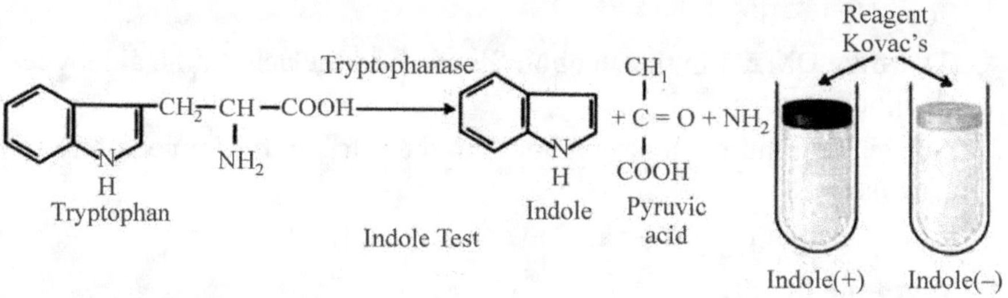

Requirements:

Nutrient broth cultures of *Escherichia coli*

1% Tryptone broth tubes

Kovac's reagent

Inoculating needle

1 mL Pipette

Procedure:

1. Prepare 1% tryptone broth tubes and sterilize the tubes in autoclave at 121°C for 15 minutes.

2. Inoculate one set of tubes with test organism and maintain one set as negative control without inoculation. Inoculate one set of tubes with *Escherichia coli* to use as positive control.

3. Incubate all the tubs at 37°C for 24 hours.

4. After incubation add few drops of Kovac's reagent drop wise to all the tubes and shake gently.

5. Allow the tubes to stand for 2 minutes so that the reagent comes to the top and then compare test culture tubes with the control tubes.

Observation and results:

If Cherry red colour ring is observation at the top layer of the tube, it is positive for indole test and absence of the cherry red colour is a negative test. *E.coli* is positive for indole test.

Preparation of Kovacs Reagent:

Amyl alcohol - 150mL

p-dimethyl amino benzaldehyde (DMAB) – 10gm

Conc.HCL – 50mL

(Dissolve DMAB in the alcohol. Slowly add the acid to the aldehyde-alcohol mixture)

Store the mixture in a brown bottle in the refrigerator immediately after use)

Kovacs reagent is also available commercially

1. Tryptone broth:

Tryptone   -   10g

Sodium chloride   -   5g

Distilled water   -   1000mL

Alternate media for detecting Indole Production:

2. Tryptone peptone broth:

Casein peptone   -   10g

Sodium chloride   -   5g

Tryptone   -   5g

Distilled water   -   1000mL

28

Methyl Red and Voges-Proskauer Test (MR-VP Test)

Methyl red and Voges-Proskauer are two tests performed together on the same medium useful in separating members of the family Enterobacteriaceae. They are used to distinguish bacteria that produce a large amount of acids and those that produce neutral product acetoin (acetyl methyl carbinol) as the end product of fermenting glucose. Opposite results are usually obtained for methyl red and Voges-Proskauer test. Organisms that ferment glucose release large amount of organic acids into the medium which can be detected on addition of pH indicator Methyl Red. The organisms which produce acetoin as the end product can be detected by addition of alpha-naphthol and KOH solutions which turns the medium pink.

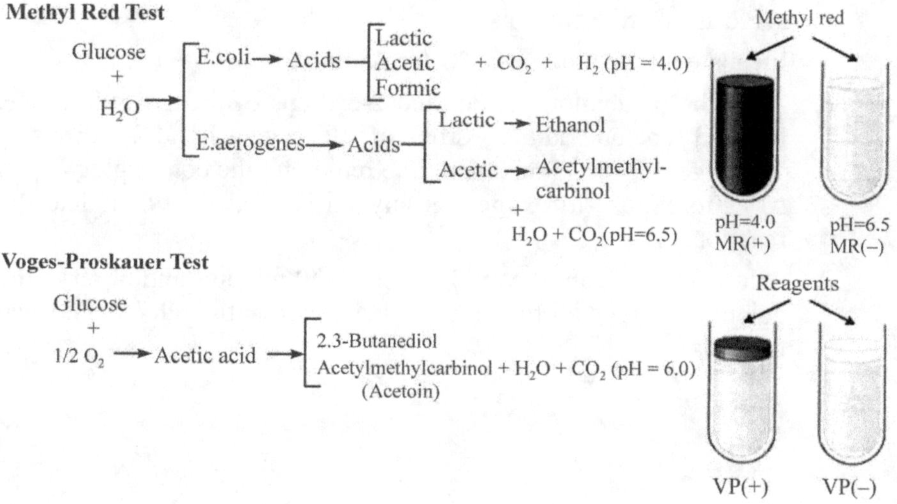

Requirements:

24 hours broth cultures of *Escherichia coli* and *Enterobacter aerogens* for positive control

MR-VP broth

Methyl red pH indicator

Voges Proskauer reagent-I (5% alpha naphthol solution in ethyl alcohol)

Voges Proskauer reagent-II (40% KOH)

Sterile test tubes

Inoculation loop

Procedure:

1. Prepare MR-VP broth and distribute 2-3 mL in 12 test tubes and sterilize at 15lbs pressure for 15 minutes.

2. Label six tubes as MR for methyl red test and six tubes as VP for Voges Proskauer test.

3. Inoculate two MR and VP labelled tubes with test bacterial culture.

4. Maintain two MR and VP labelled tubes as –ve control without inoculation and inoculate two MR labelled tubes with *Escherichia coli* and two VP labelled tubes with *Enterobacter aerogens* to serve as positive controls.

5. Incubate all the tubes at 30°C for 48 hrs.

6. After the incubation period, add 2-3 drops of methyl red on MR labelled tube and add 2-5 drops of VP reagent I and 2-5 drops of VP reagent II on VP labelled tube removing the cotton plugs open so as to expose to oxygen as oxygen is needed to complete the reaction.

7. Allow the reaction to complete for 15-30 minutes and observe the colour change in all the tubes and compare with both –ve and +ve controls.

Observation and results:

1. **Methyl Red test**: On addition of methyl red, if the colour of the medium changes to red it is positive for MR test, while if colour of the medium decolourized and turns yellow indicating negative for MR test. *E.coli* is positive for methyl red test.

2. **Voges Proskauer test**: On addition of VP-I and VP-II reagents, if colour of the medium changes to crimson to ruby pink the test is positive and if no colour change is observed indicative of negative test. *Enterobacter aerogens* is +ve for VP test.

Precautions:

1. The VP test should be done at 48 hours. Longer incubation times could result in false positives.

2. The VP reagents must be added in the order listed and with mixing to avoid weak-positive or false negative results.

3. The broth must be incubated for a minimum of 48 hours for the MR test.

4. Results of the MR and VP tests need to be used in conjugation with other biochemical tests to differentiate genus and species with in Enterobacteriaceae.

MRVP broth (glucose phosphate broth):

Peptone 7g

Dextrose -5g

Dipotassium phosphate-5g

Distilled water -1000mL

Citrate Test

Citrate test is useful in differentiating enteric bacteria on the basis of their ability to use citrate as a sole carbon source. When bacteria metabolize citrate, CO_2 is liberated and combines with sodium (supplied by sodium citrate) and forms sodium carbonate, an alkaline product in the medium. The shift in the pH turns bromothymol blue indicator in the medium from green to blue above pH 7.6. The organism which is positive for this test changes the colour of the medium from green to blue.

Citrate Test

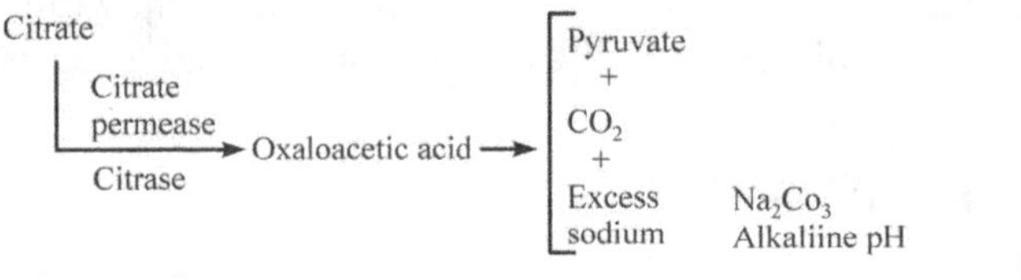

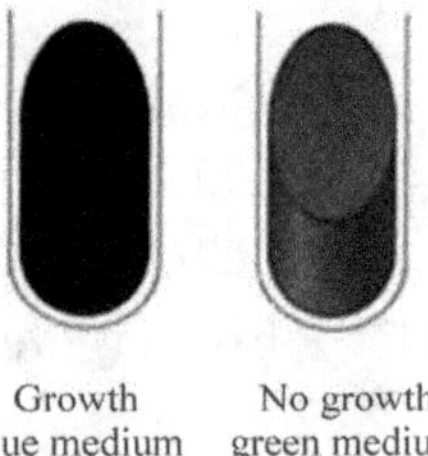

Citrate test

Requirements:

Simmon's citrate agar medium

Autoclave

24 hours culture of *E.coli*

Inoculation loop

Procedure:

1. Prepare the Simmon's citrate agar medium and adjust the pH to 6.9 and sterilize at 15lbs pressure for 15min and prepare 6 slants.

2. Inoculate one set of slants with test organism by streaking on the agar surface of the slant and maintain one set as negative control without any inoculation and inoculate one set with *E.coli* so as to use as positive control.

3. Incubate all the tubes at 37°C for 24 to 48hrs.

4. At the end of incubation period compare the test culture tube with positive and negative control tubes for change in colour.

Observation and Results:

If colourof the medium changes to blue it is citrate positive. *E.coli* is citrate positive.

Simmon's Citrate agar (pH 6.9)

Ammonium dihydrogen phosphate	1.0g
Dipotassium phosphate	1.0g
Sodium chloride	2.0g
Magnesium sulphate	0.2g
Agar	15g
Bromo thymol blue	0.08mL
Distilled water	1000mL

30

Carbohydrate Fermentation Test

The carbohydrate fermentation test is used to determine whether bacteria can ferment a specific carbohydrate or not. This fermentation pattern is useful in differentiating bacterial species. Basal medium containing a single carbohydrate such as glucose, lactose, sucrose or any other carbohydrate is used for this purpose. Microorganisms metabolize these carbohydrates to meet their energy requirements resulting in the production of acids or gases. The production of acids can be detected by incorporating pH indicator in the medium (phenol red) which is red at neutral pH and turns yellow at or below pH 6.8. Production of gas can be detected by a small inverted tube called Durham tubes immersed in the medium.

Requirements:

Phenol red carbohydrate broth

Test bacterial culture

Cultures of *Escherichia coli*

Sterile Durham's tubes

Procedure:

1. Prepare phenol red with glucose broth medium and distribute 5.0mLeach in 6 test tubes with Durham's tube inserted upside down and sterilize at 121°C for 15 minutes at 15lbs pressure.

2. After sterilization allow the medium to cool and inoculate one set of tubes with test bacterial culture, one set of tubes are maintained as a negative control without any inoculation and inoculate one set with *E.coli* to serve as positive control.

3. Incubate all the inoculated tubes at 37°C for 24 hrs.

Observation and results: Observe the changes in inoculated and uninoculated tubes. Colour change to yellow in media indicates acid production and accumulation of gas in Durham's tubes indicates gas production.

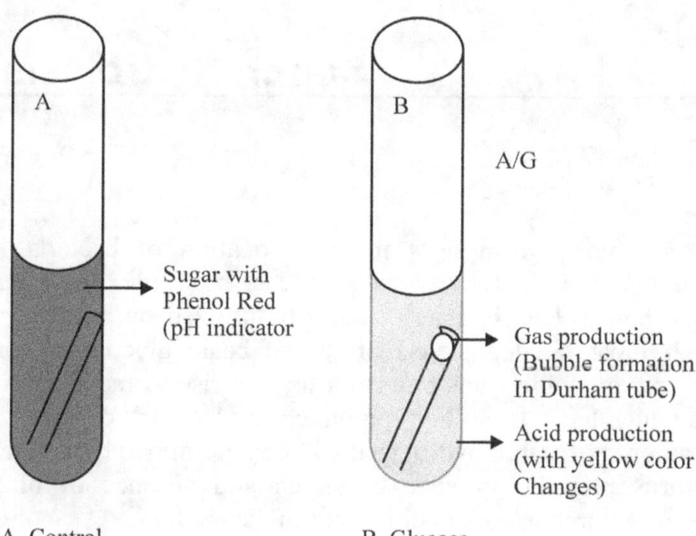

Phenol red carbohydrate broth:

(Carbon source may vary depending upon test requirement)

Peptone	10.0g
Carbohydrate	5.0g
Sodium chloride	5.0g
Phenol red	0.01g
Distilled water	1000mL
pH	7.3

31

Starch Hydrolysis Test

One of the biochemical tests for identification of bacteria is starch hydrolysis test. Starch is a polymer of glucose molecule linked together by glycosidic bonds. Hence, starch cannot be utilized by bacterial cells for energy. It must be degraded first to the basic glucose by producing amylase enzyme which acts on starch to give rise to maltose or glucose. Bacteria which have the ability to produce amylase will degrade the starch and the amount of starch hydrolyzed will be determined by iodine reagent. Iodine turns blue in presence of starch and absence of blue colour indicates that starch is no longer present in the medium.

Requirements:

Nutrient agar medium with 1% soluble starch

Test bacterial culture

Petri plates

Bacillus subtilis

Inoculating loop

Laminar air flow

Grams iodine

Dropper

Procedure:

1. Weigh 1.0 gram of starch and add to small amount of distilled water and boil for ten minutes with constant stirring until it is soluble and then add it to nutrient agar medium and makeup to 100mL.

2. Sterilize the medium at 121°C for 15 minutes.

3. After sterilization allow the medium to cool and pour approximately 20mL into Petri plates and allow it to solidify.

4. Following aseptic conditions, streak the test bacterial culture on the surface of the agar medium in the plate with the help of inoculation needle.

5. Maintain one plate as a negative control without inoculation and one as a positive control by inoculating with *Bacillus subtilis*.

6. Now incubate both the test and control plates at 37°C for 24-48 hours.

7. At the end of incubation period flood the plates with Grams iodine solution and wait for 5 minutes.

8. Measure the decolourised area around the bacterial culture.

Observations and Results:

Upon addition of iodine solution, a clear zone around the growth of the bacterial culture indicates hydrolysis of starch and blue colour indicates non-hydrolysis of starch. *Bacillus subtilis* is starch hydrolysis test positive

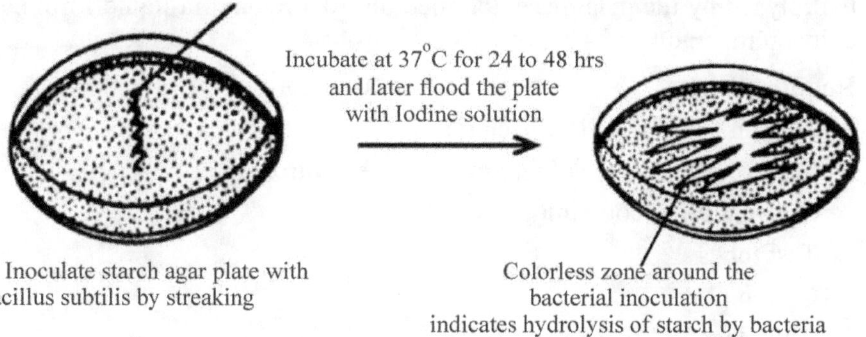

Inoculate starch agar plate with
Bacillus subtilis by streaking

Colorless zone around the
bacterial inoculation
indicates hydrolysis of starch by bacteria

Hydrolysis of starch by Bacteria

32

Gelatin Hydrolysis Test

Gelatin is a protein produced by hydrolysis of collagen which is a major component of connective tissues found in the human being and other animals. Gelatin hydrolysis test is used to find the ability of a bacterial culture to produce gelatinase, a proteolytic enzyme that liquefies gelatin and liberate amino acids. The bacteria can take up these amino acids and use them in their metabolic process. Gelatin exists as a liquid above 25°C and solidifies when cooled below 25°C. Once the gelatin has been hydrolysed by the gelatinase, the medium will remain in liquid form even at low temperature of 4°C.

Requirements:

24 hours culture of test bacteria

Culture of *Bacillus subtilis* for positive control

Nutrient broth containing 4% gelatin

Test tubes

Cotton plugs

Autoclave

Inoculating needle

Laminar air flow

Procedure:

1. Prepare nutrient agar medium with gelatin and distribute in 6.0 test tubes and sterilize at 121°C for 15 minutes.

2. Prepare agar deep tubes by keeping them in vertical position in the test tube stand.

3. Inoculate a set of nutrient gelatin stabs from top to bottom with test bacterial culture by puncturing with a straight needle and by withdrawing the needle through the same path.

4. Maintain one set as a negative control without bacterial inoculation and one set as positive control by stab inoculation of *Bacillus subtilis*.

5. Incubate all the inoculated and uninoculated nutrient gelatin stab tubes at 37°C for 24-48hrs.

6. After incubation period, place the control and inoculated tubes in ice bath or refrigerator at 4°C.

7. Examine the chilled tubes whether the medium is in liquid or solid form.

Observation and results:

Positive test:

Inoculated tubes that remain liquified even after chilling indicate the hydrolysis of gelatin by production of gelatinase enzyme by inoculated bacteria. *Bacillus subtilis* is positive for gelatin liquification test.

Negative test:

Inoculated tubes that remain solid even after chilling indicates a negative test. The medium in negative control remains in solid state at chilling temperature.

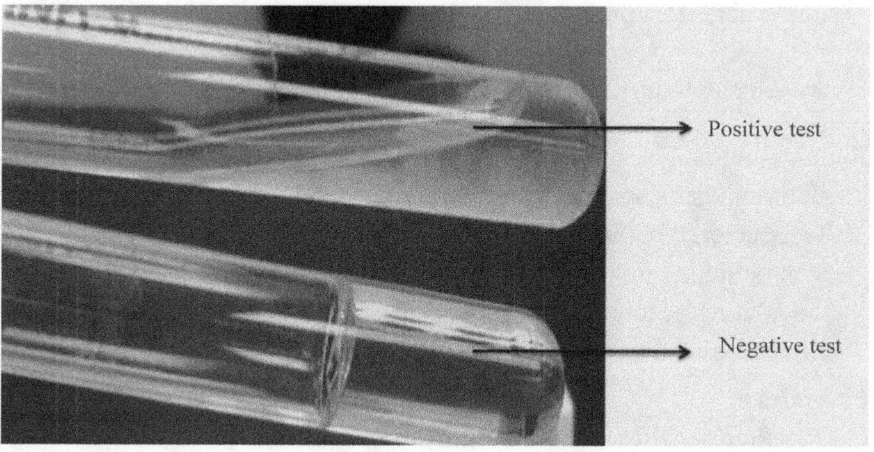

33

H₂S Production Test

This test is used to find the ability of a bacterial culture to reduce sulphur containing compounds to sulfides. This is mainly used in identification of members of the family Enterobacteriaceae and occasionally other bacteria. Sulphide indole motility agar medium (SIM) is used for this test which contains peptone (Cysteine) and sodium thiosulphate ($Na_2S_2O_3$) as substrate and ferrous ammonium sulphate as H_2S indicator. Hydrogen sulphide is liberated through the reduction of sulphur containing amino acids (cystine, cysteine and methionine) which results from the decomposition of proteins by bacteria. The hydrogen sulphide thus liberated reacts with metal salts ($FeSO_4$) forming a visible insoluble black ferrous sulphide precipitate.

Amino acids (Sulphur containing) ⟶ Pyruvic acids + ammonia + hydrogen sulphide

Hydrogen sulphide + ferrous sulphate ⟶ ferrous sulphide + Sulphuric acid.

Requirements:

Nutrient agar slants of *Proteus vulgaris*

Test bacterial culture

SIM (sulphide indole motility) agar medium,

Inoculating needle,

Laminar air flow.

Procedure:

1. Prepare SIM agar medium and distribute in to test tubes and sterilize at 121°C for 15 minutes at 15lbs pressure.

2. Prepare the stabs and label them properly. Inoculate one set with test bacteria by stab inoculation using inoculation needle and one set with *Proteus vulgaris* which is positive control and maintain one set as negative control without inoculation.

3. Incubate the control and inoculated tubes at 25°C for 48 hrs.

4. After incubation, observe the tubes for colour change along the stab by comparing with controls.

Observation and results:

Appearance of 'black colour along the line of the stab inoculation indicates the production of hydrogen sulphide. *Proteus vulgaris* is H₂S test positive.

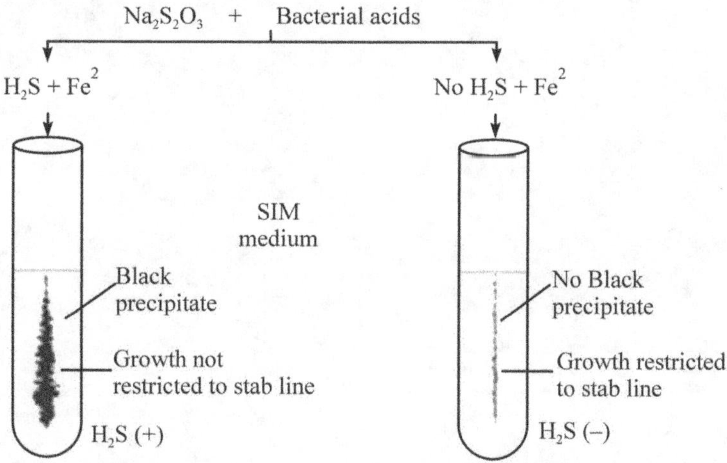

Detection of Hydrogen sulfide Production

SIM (sulphide indole motility) agar medium

Peptone-30g

Beef extract-3.0g

Ferrous ammonium sulphate-0.2g

Sodium thiosulphate-0.025g

Agar-2g

pH-7.3

Note: This medium can also be used for demonstration of bacterial motility.

Bacterial Motility

34

Wet Mount Method

Determination of Bacterial Motility

Some bacteria possess extremely thin hair-like appendages called flagella which are the organs of locomotion. Bacteria which possess flagella have the intrinsic ability to move in the surrounding medium and the bacteria which don't have flagella remains suspended in a non-motile state. Bacterial motility can be determined by microscopic and macroscopic methods.

I. Methods for working with non pathogens
   A. Wet mount slide
   B. Hanging drop method

II. Methods for working with pathogens
   A. Soft agar and
   B. Deep tube method

A. Wet mount slide

Requirements

24 hours bacterial culture of *Proteus vulgaris*

Glass slide

Cover slip

Inoculating needle

Bunsen burner

Procedure:

1. Take a clean grease free glass slide, by following aseptic technique place a drop of bacterial culture on the slide.

2. Cover the culture drop with a cover slip with the help of a needle and observe under the microscope at low power followed by high power objective lens.

Precautions:

1. Place the cover slip gently over the drop of bacteria, if not bacteria are pressed between the flat surface of slide and the cover slip.
2. Observe the slide quickly under the microscope.

Advantages:

1. Simplest and easiest way to determine bacterial motility.
2. Natural shape, size and arrangement can be observed in live condition.
3. Require no special slide

Disadvantages:

1. The rate of bacterial movement slows down because the wet mount slide dries due to the heat from the light of microscope.

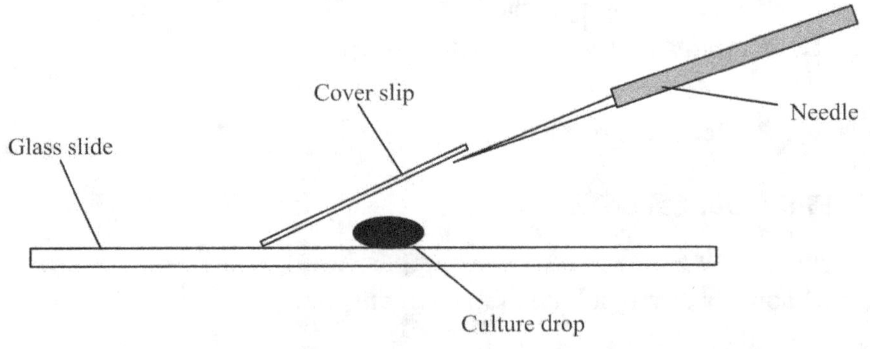

Wet mount

35

Hanging Drop Method

Hanging drop preparation is a useful technique for microscopic examination of bacteria without staining. In this technique, a drop of bacterial culture is placed on a coverslip and the drop is inverted over the cavity of a special slide called cavity slide so that the drop hangs in the cavity, the petroleum jelly forms a seal that prevents evaporation. This preparation gives a good view of microbial motility.

Materials Required:

Cavity slide,

Cover slip,

Petroleum jelly or Vaseline,

Match sticks

24-hour old broth culture of bacteria *Proteus vulgaris*

Inoculation loop and

Microscope (compound, dark-field or phase contrast).

Immersion oil,

Procedure:

1. A cavity slide is taken and cleaned properly under running tap water, such that water does not remain as drops on its surface.

2. The slide is dried by wiping with filter paper and subsequently, moving it over the flame.

3. A ring of petroleum jelly (or Vaseline) is applied around the cavity with a match stick.

4. With the help of sterilized inoculation loop, a small drop of the bacterial suspension is placed at the center of a coverslip.

5. The cavity slide is inverted and placed on the coverslip, in such a way that, the drop is in the center of the cavity.

6. The slide and coverslip are pressed together gently so that the cavity is sealed with petroleum jelly. Care should be taken to see that no part of the cavity touches the drop.

7. The slide is inverted quickly, such that the drop hangs into the cavity without touching it.

8. Clip the slide on the microscope stage, focus on low power (10X) and look through the eyepiece. Raise the objective lens slowly using coarse adjustment knob until the edge of the drop is observed as an irregular line crossing the field.

9. After focusing the edge look at each side for motility of the bacteria. For clear visibility use fine adjustment knob.

10. Adjust the light using diaphragm level to maximize the visibility of bacterial motility.

11. Now when motility is clearly observed, without disturbing the focus, turn to high power (40X) lens to observe clear magnified motile bacterial cells.

12. As the drop hangs, it thins towards the edge, for which the edge contains less number of bacteria to be observed clearly for motility.

13. Usually, aerobic bacteria come towards the edge to get more oxygen for respiration, for which they can be observed on the edge.

14. Without disturbing the focus remove the slide and place a drop of immersion oil on the coverslip just above the hanging drop and the edge of the hanging drop is observed under 100X objective lens.

Observation and Results:

Rod shaped extremely motile *Proteus vulgaris* will be seen under microscope.

Precautions:

1. The broth culture should not be more than 24 hours old as bacteria loose motility as they grow older.

2. Place only a micro drop of bacterial culture on the cover slip.

3. Do not apply more Vaseline around the cavity.

4. Observe motility of the bacteria immediately after preparation of the slide if not motility may not be seen.

5. The slide and cover slip should be sterilized after examination is over.

6. The depression slide should be inverted over the cover slip in such a way that the suspension does not touch the surface of the concavity at any point.

Advantages:

1. Easy to prepare within a short time.

2. Live bacterial motility can be seen.

Disadvantages:

1. Risky to use with highly pathogenic organisms.

Cavity slide:

1. These slides are useful as moist chambers for observing hanging drops.

2. The slides have polished round depressions 15mm in diameter and 1mm deep.

3. Available with either one or two or three depressions (cavities) of dimensions: 76 x 25 x 1.25mm.

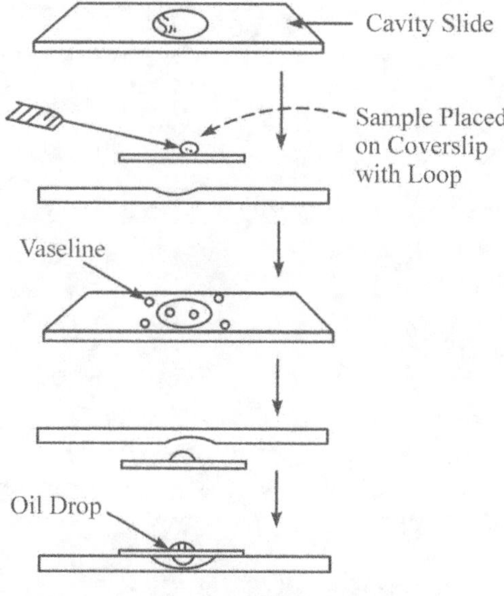

Hanging drop preparation

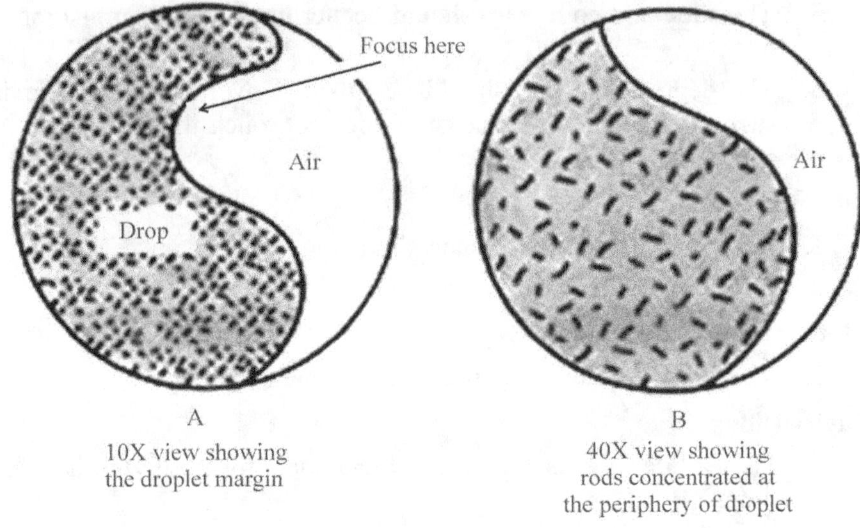

Examination of hanging drop under the microscope

36

Soft Agar and Agar Deep Tube Methods

Motile bacteria are able to move through agar in chase of nutrients. If a drop of bacterial culture is placed in the center of an agar plate and the plate is incubated, the bacteria start to move out of the center. At a distance from the center, bacteria divide and the progeny continues to move out. This causes the formation of concentric rings called swarms on the surface of agar which can be easily recognized by the naked eye.

Requirements:

Trypticase soy agar plates,

24 hrs old culture of *Proteus mirabilis* and *Staphylococcus epidermis*

Bunsen burner

Incubator

a. Motility test with soft agar plates:

1. Prepare trypticase -soy agar plates and label properly using glass marker.

2. Following aseptic technique, inoculate the culture of *Proteus mirabilis* as a spot about 5mm in diameter at the centre of the plate on the surface of agar.

3. Main one plate as control by inoculating with *Staphylococcus epidermis*.

4. Incubate the plates at 37°C for 24-48hrs.

5. Observe the plates after incubation period.

Observation:

Motile Bacteria: At the end of incubation period *Proteus mirabilis* inoculated plate will be seen covered with culture due to its rapid spread on the surface.

Non-motile Bacteria: The plate inoculated with *S.epidermis* will be seen with discrete and restricted growth.

Advantages:

1. Safe technique when testing motility of pathogens.

2. No need of microscope.

b. Motility test with agar deep tubes:

Requirements:

SIM (Sulphide Indole Motility medium) stabs

Inoculation needle

Bunsen burner

Incubator

Procedure:

1. Prepare SIM agar tubes and inoculate separately with *P. mirabilis* and *S. epidermis* by stab inoculation.

2. Keep "Sham" inoculate soft agar deep to serve as uninoculated control.

3. This is done stabbing sterile soft agar deep tubes with sterile needle. This type of control tube will help us to determine the difference between disturbed agar and growth of non-motile cultures after inoculation.

4. Incubate the inoculated tubes at 37°C for 24 hrs.

5. Observe the tubes after 24-36 hours of incubation by holding up to the light.

Observation and results:

Motile Bacteria: The tube inoculated with *P. mirabilis* shows diffuse, hazy growth that spread throughout the medium rendering it slightly opaque.

Non-motile Bacteria: The tube inoculated with *S. epidermis* shows growth confined to the stab line, have sharply defined margins and leave the surrounding medium clearly transparent.

Advantages:

1. This technique is useful in determining highly pathogenic bacteria.
2. This technique takes longer time than wet mount and hanging drop methods.
3. No need of microscope.

Microbial Assay of Antibiotics

37

Microbial Assay of Antibiotics

The microbiological assay of an antibiotic is based upon a comparison of the inhibition of growth of micro-organisms by measured concentrations of the antibiotics under examination with that produced by known concentrations of a standard preparation of the antibiotic having a known activity.

As per Indian Pharmacopoea (1996) the microbial assay of antibiotic is carried out by two methods

- The cylinder-plate (or cup-plate) method and
- The turbidimetric (or tube assay) method.

The main steps involve in Microbial assay of antibiotics are:

1. Preparation of media
2. Preparation of standard solution
3. Preparation of buffer solution
4. Preparation of sample solution
5. Selection of test organism
6. Preparation of inoculum.
7. Determination of inoculum
8. Temperature Control
9. Adopting cylindrical or Turbidimetric method

1. Media Preparation:

Media has to be prepared according to the requirement of the specified test organism from the ingredients listed in Table 1. However, minor modifications of the individual ingredients may be made, or reconstituted dehydrated media may be used provided the resulting media have equal or better growth-promoting properties and give a similar standard curve response.

Method of preparation: Dissolve the ingredients in sufficient water to produce 1000 mL and add sufficient 1 M sodium hydroxide or 1 M hydrochloric acid, as required so that after sterilization the pH is as given in Table 1.

Table 1 Media: Quantities of ingredients per 1000 ml

Ingredient	Medium									
	A	**B**	**C**	**D**	**E**	**F**	**G**	**H**	**I**	**J**
Peptone	6.0	6.0	5.0	6.0	6.0	6.0	9.4	–	10.0	–
Pancreatic digest of casein	4.0	–	–	4.0	–	–	–	17.0	–	15.0
Yeast extract	3.0	3.0	1.5	3.0	3.0	3.0	4.7	–	–	–
Beef extract	1.5	1.5	1.5	1.5	1.5	1.5	2.4	–	10.0	–
Dextrose	1.0	–	1.0	1.0	–	–	10.0	2.5	–	–
Papaic digest of soyabean	–	–	–	–	–	–	–	3.0	–	5.0
Agar	15.0	15.0		15.0	15.0	15.0	23.5	12.0	17.0	15.0
Glycerin	–	–	–	–	–	–	–	–	10.0	–
Polysorbate 80	–	–	–	–	–	–	–	10.0*	–	–
Sodium chloride	–	–	3.5	–	–	–	10.0	5.0	3.0	5.0
Dipotassium Hydrogen Phosphate	–	–	3.68	–	–	–	–	2.5	–	–
Potassium dihydrogen Phosphate	–	–	1.32	–	–	–	–	–	–	–
Final pH (after sterilization)	6.5-6.6	6.5-6.6	6.95-7.05	7.8-8.0	7.8-8.0	5.8-6.0	6.0-6.2	7.1-7.3	6.9-7.1	7.2-7.4

*Quantity in ml, to be added after boiling the media to dissolve the agar.

2. Standard Preparation and Units of Activity:

A Standard Preparation is an authentic sample of the appropriate antibiotic for which the potency has been precisely determined by reference to the appropriate international standard. The Potency of the standard preparation may be expressed in International Units or in µg per mg of the pure antibiotic.

To prepare a stock solution, dissolve a quantity of the Standard Preparation of a given antibiotic accurately weighed and previously dried where so indicated in Table 3, in the solvent specified in the table, and then dilute to the required concentration as indicated. Store in a refrigerator and use within the period indicated.

On the day of assay, prepare from the stock solution five or more test dilutions, the successive solutions increasing stepwise in concentration, usually in the ratio 1:1.25 for Method A or smaller for Method B. Use the final diluent specified and a sequence such that the middle or median has the concentration specified in Table 3.

3. **Buffer Solutions:**

Prepare buffer solutions by dissolving the following quantities given in Table 2 of dipotassiumhydrogen phosphate (K_2HPO_4) and potassium dihydrogen phosphate (KH_2PO_4)in sufficient water to produce 1000 mL after sterilization, adjusting the pH with 8 M phosphoric acid (H_3PO_4) or 10 M potassium hydroxide (KOH)

Table 2 Buffer solutions

Buffer No.	Dipotassium Hydrogen Phosphate, K_2HPO_4 (g)	Potassium Dihydrogen Phosphate, K_2HPO_4 (g)	pH adjusted after sterilization to
1	2.0	8.0	6.0 ± 0.1
2	16.73	0.523	8.0 ± 0.1
3	–	13.61	4.5 ± 0.1
4	20.0	80.00	6.0 ± 0.1
5	35.0	–	10.5 ± 0.1*
6	13.6	4.0	7.0 ± 0.2

*After addition of 2 ml of 10M potassium hydroxide

4. **Preparation of the Sample Solution:**

From the information available for the substance under examination (the "unknown"), assign to it an assumed potency per unit weight or volume, and on this assumption prepare on the day of the assay a stock solution and test dilution as specified for each antibiotic in Table 3 but with the same final diluent as used for the Standard Preparation. The assay with 5 levels of the Standard requires only one level of the unknown at a concentration assumed equal to the median level of the standard.

5. **Test Organisms:**

The test organism for each antibiotic is selected as per table Table 4, together with its identification number in the American Type

Culture Collection (ATCC). Maintain a culture on slants of the medium and under the incubation conditions specified in Table 5, and transfer weekly to fresh slants

Table 3 Test organisms for Microbiological assay of antibiotics

Antibiotic	Test Organism	ATTC No.
Amikacin	*Staphylococcus aureus*	29737
Amphotericin B	*Saccharomyces cerevisiae*	9763
Bacitracin	*Micrococcus luteus*	10240
Bleomycin	*Mycobacterium smegmatis*	607
Carbenicillin	*Pseudomonas aeruginosa*	25619
Doxycyclin	*Bacillus pumilus*	14884
Erythromycin	*Micrococcus luteus*	9341
Framycetin	*Bacillus pumilus*	14884
	Bacillus subtilis	6633
Gentamycin	*Staphylococcus epidermidis*	12228
Kanamycin sulphate	*Bacillus pumilus*	14884
Neomycin	*Staphylococcus epidermidis*	12228
Novobiocin	*Staphylococcus epidermidis*	12228
Nystatin	*Saccharomyces cerevisiae*	2601
Oxytetracyclin	*Bacillus cereus var mycoides*	11778
	Staphylococcus aureus	29737
Polymyxin B	*Bordetella bronchiseptica*	4617
Rifampicin	*Bacillus subtilis*	6633
Streptomycin	*Bacillus subtilis*	6633
	Klebsiella pneumoniae	10031
Tetracycline	*Bacillus cereus*	11778
	Staphylococcus aureus	29737

ATTC = American Type Culture Collection

[Adapted From : **Indian Pharmacopoea,** Vol. II, 1996]

6.   Preparation of Inoculums:

Prepare the microbial suspensions for the inoculum for the assay as given in Table 5. If the suspensions are prepared by these methods, growth characteristics are sufficiently uniform so that the inoculum can be adequately determined.

Table 4 Stock solutions and test dilutions of standard preparation

Antibiotic (1)	Assay Method (2)	Prior Drying (3)	Initial solvent (further diluents, if different) (4)	Final Stock Concentration Per ml (5)	Use before (number of days) (6)	Final diluent (7)	Median dose µg or units per ml (8)	Incubation Temp (°C) (9)
Amikacin	B	No	water	1mg	14	Water	10 µg	32-35
Amphotericin B	A	Yes	DMF[7]	1mg	Same day	B5	1.0 µg	29-31
Bacitracin	A	Yes	0.01 M HCl	100 units	Same day	B1	1.0 Unit	32-35
Bleomycin	A	Yes	B6[8]	2 Units	14	B6	0.04 Unit	32-35
Carbenicillin	A	No	Bl	1 mg	14	B6	20 µg	36-37.5
Doxycyclin	B	No	0.01M HCl	1mg	5	Water	0.1 µg	35-37
Erythromycin	A	Yes	Methanol 10mg/ml)[8] (B2)	1 mg	14	B2	1.0 µg	35-37
Framycetin	A	Yes	B2	1 mg	14	B2	1.0 µg	30-35
Gentamycin	A	Yes	B2	1 mg	30	B2	0.1 µg	36-37.5
Kannamycin sulphate	A[1]	No	B2	800 units	30	B2	0.8 Unit	37-39
Kanamycin B	A	No	B2	1000 units	30	B2	1.0 Unit	32-35
Neomycin	A	Yes	B2	1 mg	14	B2	1.0 µg	36-37.5
Novobiocin	A	Yes	Ethanol (10mg/ml)[9],(B2)	1 mg	5	B4	0.5 µg	32-35
Nystatin	A	Yes	DMF[7]	1000 units	Same day	B4	20 units	35-39
Oxytetracycline	A[3]	No	0.1M HCl	1 mg	4	B3	2.5µg	32-35
	B[2]	No	0.1M HCl	1 mg	4	Water	0.24 µg	35-39
Polymyxin B	A	Yes	Water, (B4)	10,000 Units	14	B4	10 Units	35-39
Rifampicin	A	No	Methanol	1 mg	1	B1	5.0 µg	29-31
Streptomycin	A[4]	Yes	Water	1 mg	30	water	1.0 µg	32-35
	B[5]	Yes	water	1 mg	30	water	30 µg	32-37
Tetracycline	A[3]	No	0.1M HCl	1 mg	1	water	2.5 µg	32-35
	B[6]	No	0.1M HCl	1 mg	4	water	0.24 µg	35-37

1. With *Bacillus pumilis ATCC* 14884 as test organism, 2. With *Staphylococcus aureus* ATCC 29737 as test organism;3.With *Bacillus cereus* or *mycoides* ATTC 11778 as test organism; 4.With *Bacillus subtilis* ATCC6633 as test organism; 5.With *Klebsiella pneumonia* ATCC 10031 as test organism; 6. With *Staphylococcus aureus* ATCC 29737 as test organism; 7.DMF=Dimethylformamide; 8. In columns 4 and 7, B denotes buffer solution and the number following refers to the buffer number in table. Initial concentration of stock solution.

Notes-For Amphotericin B and Nystatin, prepare the standard solutions and the sample test solution simultaneous.

For Amphotericin B, further dilute the stock solution with dimethyl formamide to give concentrations of 12.8,16,20,25 and 31.2 µg per ml prior to making the test solutions.The test diluton of the sample prepared from the solution of the substance being examined should contain the same amount of dimethyl formamid as the test dilutions of the Standard Preparation.

For Bacitracin, each of the standard test dilutions should contain the same amount of hydrochloric acid as the test dilution of the sample.

For Nystatin, further dilute the stock solution with dimethylformamide to give concentrations of 64.0, 80.0, 100.0, 125.0 and 156.0 µg per ml prior to making the test dilutions. Prepare the standard response line solutions simultaneously with dilutions of the sample being examined. The test dilutions of the sample prepared from the solution of the substance being examined should contain the same amount of dimethylformamide as the test dilutions of the Standard Preparations. Protect the solutions from light.

When making the stock solution of Polymixin B, add 2 ml of water for each 5 mg of the weighed Standard preparation material.

Where indicated, dry about 100 mg of the Standard Preparation before use in an oven at a pressure not exceeding 0.7k pa at 60°C for 3 hours, except in the fine of Bleomycin (dry at 25°C for 4 hours). Novobiocin (dry at 100°C for 4 hours),Gentamycin (dry at 110° for 3 hours) and Nystatin (dry at 40°C for 2 hours).

When two level factorial assays are performed use the following test doses per ml; Amphotericin B,1.0 to 4.0µg;Bacitracin,1.0 to 4.0 Units; Kanamycin Sulphate ,5.0 to 20.0 units;Streptomycin,5.0 to 20.0 µg.

[Adapted From: Indian Pharmacopoea Vol. II 1996]

Table 5 Preparation of inoculum

S.No	Test organism	Incubation conditions			Suggested dilution factor	Suggested inoculum composition		
		Medium/ Method of preparation	Temp (°C)	Time		Medium	Amount (ml per 100ml)	Antibiotics assayed
1.	*Bacillus cereus Var.mycoides*	$A^{1/2}$	32-35	5 days	-	F	As required	Oxytetracycline Tetracycline
2.	*Bacillus pumilus*	$A^{1/2}$	32-35	5 days	-	D	As required	Framycetin Kanamycin sulphate
3	*Bacillus subtilis*	$A^{1/2}$	32-35	5 days	-	E E B	As required As required As required	Framycetin Kanamycin B Rifampicin
4	*Bordetella bronchiseptica*	A/1	32-35	24 hr	1:20	H	0.1	Polymyxin B
5	*Klebsiella pneumoniae*	A/1	36-37	24 hr	1:25	C	0.1	Streptomycin
6	*Micrococcus luteus (9341)*	A/1	32-35	24 hr	1:40	D	1.5	Erythromycin
7	*Micrococcus luteus (10240)*	A/1	32-35	24 hr	1:35	A	0.3	Bacitracin
8	*Mycobacterium smegmatis*	J/4	36-37.5	48 hr	As determined	I	1.0	Bleomycin
9	*Pseudomonas aeruginosa[2]*	A/1	36-37.5	24 hr	1:25	H	0.5	Carbenicillin
10	*Saccharomyces cerevisiae (9363)*	G/3	29-31	48 hr	As determined	G	1.0	Amphotericin B
11	*Saccharomyces cerevisiae (2601)*	G/3	29/31	48 hr	As determined	G	1.0	Nystatin

Table 5 *Contd….*

S.No	Test organism	Incubation conditions			Suggested dilution factor	Suggested inoculum composition		
		Medium/ Method of preparation	Temp (°C)	Time		Medium	Amount (ml per 100ml)	Antibiotics assayed
12	*Staphylococcus aureus*	A/1	32-35	24 hr	1:20	C	0.1	Amikacin
								Doxycycline
								Oxytetracycline
								Tetracycline
						C	0.2	Kanamycin sulphate
13	*Staphylococcus epidermidis*	A/1	32-35	24 hr	1:40	D	0.03	Gentamycin
						D	0.4	Neomycin
						A	4.0	Novobiocin

1. Use Medium A containing 300 mg of mamganese sulphate per litre

2. For Pseudomonas aeruginosa in the assay of carbenicillin, use the dilution yielding 25% light transmission, rather than the stock suspension, for preparing the inoculum suspension.

Methods of preparation of test organism suspension

1. Maintain the test organism on slants of Medium A and transfer to a fresh slant once a week .Incubate the slants at the temperature indicated above for 24 hours. Using 3 ml of saline solution, wash the organism from the agar slant onto a large agar surface of Medium A such as a Roux bottle containing 250 ml of agar .Incubate for 24 hours at the appropriate temperature. Wash the growth from the nutrient surface using 50 ml of saline solution. Store the test organism under refrigerator. Determine the amount of suspensions to be added to each 100 ml of agar of nutrient broth by use of test plates or test broth. Store the suspension under refrigerator.

2. Proced as described under Method 1 but incubate the Roux bottle for 5 days. Centrifuge and decant the supernatane liquid. Resuspend the sediment with 50 to 70 ml of saline solution and heat the suspension for 30 minutes at 70°. Wash the spore suspension three times with 50 to 70 ml of *saline solution.* Resuspend in 50 to 70 ml of *saline solution* and heat-shock again for 30 minutes. Use test plates to determine the amount of the suspension required for 100 ml of agar. Store the suspension under refrigeration.

3. Maintain the test organism on 10 ml agar slants of Medium G. Incubate at 32° to 35° for 24 hours. Inoculate 100 ml of nutrient broth. Incubate for 16 to 18 hours at 37° and proceed as described in Method 1.

4. Proceed as described in Method 1 but wash the growth from the nutrient surface using 50 ml of Medium 1 (prepared without agar) in place of *saline solution.* [Adapted From : **Indian Pharmacopoea,** Vol. II, 1996]

7. **Determination of Inoculum:**

   a. **For Method A**.

   After the suspension is prepared as given under Table 5, add different volumes of it to each of several different flasks containing 100 mL of the medium specified in Table 3 (the volume of suspension suggested in Table 3 may be used as a guide). Using these inocula, prepare inoculated plates as described for the specific antibiotic assay. While conducting cylinder-plate assays, double-layer plates may be prepared by pouring a seed layer (inoculated with the desired micro organism) over a solidified uninoculated base layer. For each Petri dish, 21 mL of base layer and 4 mL of the seed layer may be generally suitable. Fill each cylinder with the median concentration of the antibiotic (Table 3) and then incubate the plates. After incubation, examine and measure the zones of inhibition. The volume of suspension that produces the optimum zones of inhibition with respect to both clarity and diameter determines the inoculum to be used for the assay.

   b. **For Method B**.

   Proceed as described for Method A and, using the several inocula, carry out the procedure as described for the specific antibiotic assay running only the high and low concentrations of the standard response curve. After incubation, read the absorbances of the appropriate tubes. Determine which inoculum produces the best response between the low and high antibiotic concentrations and use this inoculum for the assay.

8. **Temperature Control**:

   Thermostatic control is required at several stages of a microbial assay, when culturing a microorganism and preparing its inoculum and during incubation in a plate assay. Closer control of the temperature is imperative during incubation in a tube assay which may be achieved by either circulated air or water, the greater heat capacity of water lending it some advantage over circulating air.

Spectrophotometer

Measuring transmittance within a fairly narrow frequency band requires a suitable spectrophotometer in which the wavelength of the light source can be varied or restricted by the use of a 580-nm filter for preparing inocula of the required density or with a 530-nm filter for reading an absorbance in a tube assay. For the latter purpose, the instrument may be arranged to accept the tube in which incubation takes place, to accept a modified cell fitted with a drain that facilitates rapid change of contents, or preferably fixed with a flow-through cell for a continuous flow-through analysis. Set the instrument at zero absorbance with clear, uninoculated broth prepared as specified for the particular antibiotic, including the same amount of test solution and formaldehyde as found in each sample.

Cylinder-plate assay receptacles

Use rectangular glass trays or glass or plastic Petri dishes (approximately 20 x 100 mm) having covers of suitable material and assay cylinders made of glass, porcelain, aluminium or stainless steel with outside diameter 8 mm ± 0.1 mm, inside diameter 6mm ± 0.1mm and length 10 mm ± 0.1 mm. Instead of cylinders, holes 5 to 8 mm in diameter may be bored in the medium with a sterile borer, or paper discs of suitable quality paper may be used. Carefully clean the cylinder to remove all residues. An occasional acidbath, e.g. with about *2 M nitric acid* or with *chromic acid solution* is needed.

Turbidimetric assay receptacles

For assay tubes, use glass or plastic test-tubes, e.g. 16 mm x 125 mm or 18 mm x 150 mm that are relatively uniform in length, diameter, and thickness and substantially free from surface blemishes and scratches. Cleanse thoroughly to remove all antibiotic residues and traces of cleaning solution and sterilise tubes that have been used previously before subsequent use.

Assay Designs:

a. Microbial assays gain markedly in precision by the segregation of relatively large sources of potential error and bias through suitable experimental designs. In a cylinder plate assay, the essential comparisons are restricted to relationships between zone diameter measurements within plates, exclusive of the variation between plates in their preparation and subsequent handling.

   To conduct a turbidimetric assay so that the difference in observed turbidity will reflect the differences in the antibiotic concentration requires both greater uniformity in the environment created for the tubes through closer thermostatic control of the incubator and the avoidance of systematic bias by a random placement of replicate tubes in separate tube racks, each rack containing one complete set of treatments. The essential comparisons are then restricted to relationships between the observed turbidities within racks.

Within these restrictions, two alternative designs are recommended; i.e 3-level (or 2-level) factorial assay, or a 1- level assay with a standard curve. For a factorial assay, prepare solutions of 3 or 2 corresponding test dilutions for both the standard and the unknowns on the day of the assay, as described under Preparation of the Standard and Preparation of the samples. For a 1-level assay with a standard curve, prepare instead solutions of five test dilutions of the standard and a solution of a single median test level of the unknown as described in the same sections. Consider an assay as preliminary if its computed potency with either design is less than 60 per cent or more than 150 per cent of that assumed in preparing the stock solution of the unknown. In such a case, adjust its assumed potency accordingly and repeat the assay. Microbial determinations of potency are subject to inter-assay variables as well as intra-assay variables, so that two or more independent assays are required for a reliable estimate of the potency of a given assay preparation or unknown. Starting with separately prepared stock solutions and test dilutions of both the standard and unknown, repeat the assay of a given unknown on a different day. If the estimated potency of the second assay differs significantly, as indicated by the calculated standard error, from that of the first, conduct one or more additional assays. The combined result of a series of smaller, independent assays spread over a number of days is a more reliable estimate of potency than that from a single large assay with the same total number of plates or tubes.

9. Methods:

Microbial assay of antibiotics may be carried out by employing Method A or Method B.

A. Cylinder-plate or Cup-plate method:

Inoculate a previously liquefied medium appropriate to the assay (Tables 1 and 3) with the requisite quantity of suspension of the micro organism, add the suspension to the medium at a temperature between 40° and 50° and immediately pour the inoculated medium into the petri dishes or large rectangular plates to give a depth of 3 to 4 mm (1 to 2mm for nystatin). Ensure that the layers of medium are uniform in thickness, by placing the dishes or plates on a level surface.

Store the prepared dishes or plates in a manner so as to ensure that no significant growth or death of the test organism occurs before the dishes or plates are used and that the surface of the agar layer is dry at the time of use.

Using the appropriate buffer solutions indicated in Tables 2 and 3, prepare solutions of known concentrations of the standard preparation and solutions of the corresponding assumed of concentrations the antibiotic to be examined. Where directions have been given in the individual monograph for preparing the solutions, these should be followed, and further dilutions made with buffer solution as indicated in Table 3. Apply the solutions to the surface of the solid medium in sterile cylinders or in cavities prepared in the agar. The volume of solution added to each cylinder or cavity must be uniform and sufficient almost to fill the holes when these are used. When paper discs are used these should be sterilized by exposure of both sides under a sterilizing lamp and then impregnated with the standard solutions or the test solutions and placed on the surface of the medium. When petri dishes are used, arrange the solutions of the Standard Preparation and the antibiotic under examination on each dish so that, they alternate around the dish and so that the highest concentrations of standard and test preparations are not adjacent. When plates are used, place the solutions in a Latin square design, if the plate is a square, or if it is not, in a randomised block design. The same random design should not be used repeatedly.

Leave the dishes or plates standing for 1 to 4 hours at room temperature or at 4°, as appropriate, as a period of preincubation diffusion to minimise the effects of variation in time between the application of the different solutions. Incubate them for about 18 hours at the temperature indicated in Table 3. Accurately measure the diameters or areas of the circular inhibition zones and calculate the results.

Selection of the assay design should be based on the requirements stated in the individual monograph. Some of the usual assay designs are as follows.

A. One-level assay with standard curve

Standard Solution:

Dissolve an accurately weighed quantity of the Standard Preparation of the antibiotic, previously dried where necessary, in the solvent specified in Table 3, and then dilute to the required concentration, as indicated, to give the stock solution. Store in a refrigerator and use within the period indicated. On the day of the assay prepare from the stock solution, 5 dilution (solutions S1 to S5) representing 5 test levels of the standard and increasing stepwise in the ratio of 4:5. Use the diluent specified in Table 3 and a sequence such that the middle or median has the concentration given in the table.

Sample Solution:

From the information available for the antibiotic preparation which is being examined (the"unknown") assign to it an assumed potency per unit weight or volume and on this assumption prepare on the day of the assay a stock solution with same solvent as used for the standard. Prepare from this stock solution a dilution to a concentration equal to the median level of the standard to give the sample solution.

Method:

For preparing the standard curve, use a total of 12 Petri dishes or plates to accommodate 72 cylinders or cavities. A set of 3 plates (18 cylinders or cavities) is used for each dilution. On each of the three plates of a set fill alternate cylinders or cavities with solution S3 (representing the median concentration of the standard solution) and each of the remaining 9 cylinders or cavities with one of the other 4 dilutions of the standard solution. Repeat the process for the other 3 dilutions of the standard solution. For each unknown preparation use a set of 3 plates (18 cylinders or cavities) and fill alternate cylinders or cavities with the sample solution and each of the remaining 9 cylinders of cavities with solution S3.

Incubate the plates for about 18 hours at the specified temperature and measure the diameters or the zones of inhibition.

Estimation of potency:

Average the readings of solution S3 and the readings of the concentration tested on each sets of three plates, and average also all 36 readings of solution S3. The average of the 36 readings of solution S3 is the correction point for the curve. Correct the average value obtained for each concentration (S1, S2, S4 and S5) to the figure it would be if the readings for solution S3 for that set of three plates were the same as the correction point. Thus, in correcting the value obtained with any concentration, say S1, if the average of 36 readings of S3 is, for example, 18.0 mm and the average of the S3 concentrations on one set of three plates is 17.8 mm, the correction is + 0.2 mm. If the average reading of S1 is 16.0 mm the corrected reading of S1 is 16.2 mm. Plot these corrected values including the average of the 36 readings for solutions S3 on two-cycle semilog paper, using the concentrations in Units or μg per mL (as the ordinate logarithmic scale) and the diameter of the zones of inhibition as the abscissa. Draw the straight response line either through these points by inspection or through the points plotted for highest and lowest zone diameters obtained by means of the following expressions:

$$L = \frac{3a + 2b + c - e}{5}; \; H = \frac{3e + 2d + c - a}{5}$$

where,

L = the calculated zone diameter for the lowest concentration of the standard curve response line.

H = the calculated zone diameter for the highest concentration of the standard curve response line.

c = average zone diameter of 36 readings of the reference point standard solution.

a, b, d, e = corrected average values for the other standard solutions, lowest to highest concentrations, respectively.

Average the zone diameters for the sample solution and for solutions S3 on the plates used for the sample solution. If sample gives a large average zone size than the average of the standard (solution S3), add the difference between them to the zone size of solution S3 of the standard response line. If the average sample zone size is smaller than the standard values, subtract the difference between them from the zone size of solution S3 of the standard response line. From the response line read the concentration corresponding to these corrected values of zone sizes. From the dilution factors the potency of the sample may be calculated.

B. Two-level factorial assay:

Prepare parallel dilutions containing 2 levels of both the standard (S1 and S2) and the unknown (U1 and U2). On each of four or more plates, fill each of its four cylinders or cavities with a different test dilution, alternating standard and unknown. Keep the plates at room temperature and measure the diameters of the zones of inhibition.

Estimation of potency:

Sum the diameters of the zones of each dilution and calculate the percentage potency of the sample (in terms of the standard) from the following equation:

Per cent potency = Antilog $(2.0 + a \log I)$

Wherein, 'a' may have a positive or negative value and should be used algebraically and

Where,

$$a = \frac{U1 + U2 + S1 + S2}{U1 + U2 + S1 + S2}$$

And U1 and U2 are the sums of the zone diameters with solutions of the unknown of high and low levels.

S1 and S2 are the sums of the zone diameters with solutions of the standard of high and low levels.

I = ratio of dilutions.

If the potency of the sample is lower than 60 per cent or greater that 150 per cent of the standard, the assay is invalid and should be repeated using higher or lower dilutions of the same solution. The potency of the sample may be calculated from the Expression

$$\frac{\text{per cent potency} \times \text{assumed potency of the sample}}{100}$$

C. Other designs:

1. Factorial assay containing parallel dilution of three test levels of standard and the unknown.

2. Factorial assay using two test levels of standard and two test levels of two different unknowns.

38

Turbidimetric or Tube Assay Method

The method has the advantage of a shorter incubation period for the growth of the test organism (usually 3 to 4 hours) but the presence of solvent residues or other inhibitory substances affects this assay more than the cylinder plates assay and care should be taken to ensure freedom from such substances in the final test solutions. This method is not recommended for cloudy or turbid preparations.

Prepare five different concentrations of the standard solution for preparing the standard curve by diluting the stock solution of the Standard Preparation of the antibiotic (Table 3) and increasing stepwise in the ration 4:5. Select the median concentration (Table 3) and dilute the solution of the substance being examined (unknown) to obtain approximately this concentration. Place 1 mL of each concentration of the standard solution and of the sample solution in each of the tubes in duplicate. To each tube add 9 mL of nutrient medium (Table 3) previously seeded with the appropriate test organism (Table 3).

At the same time prepare three control tubes, one containing the inoculated culture medium (culture control), another identical with it but treated immediately with 0.5 mL of *diluteformaldehyde solution* (blank) and a third containing uninoculated culture medium.

Place all the tubes, randomly distributed or in a randomized block arrangement, in an incubator or water-bath and maintain them at the specified temperature (Table 3) for 3 to 4 hours. After incubation add 0.5 mL of *dilute formaldehyde solution* to each tube. Measure the growth of the test organism by determining the absorbance at about 530 nm of each of the solutions in the tubes against the blank.

Estimation of potency:

Plot the average absorbances for each concentration of the standard on *semi-logarithmic* paper with the absorbances on the arithmetic scale and concentrations on the logarithmic scale. Construct the best straight response line through the points either by inspection or by means of the following expressions:

$$L = \frac{3a + 2b + 2c - e}{5} \; ; \; H = \frac{3e + 2d + c - a}{5}$$

where,

L = the calculated absorbance for the lowest concentration of the standard response line.

H = the calculated absorbance for the highest concentration of the standard response line.

a, b, c, d, e = average absorbance values for each concentration of the standard response line lowest to highest respectively.

Plot the values obtained for L and H and connect the points. Average the absorbances for the sample and read the antibiotic concentration from the standard response line. Multiply the concentration by the appropriate dilution factors to obtain the antibiotic content of the sample.

Precision of Microbiological Assays:

The fiducial limits of error of the estimated potency should not be less than 95 per cent and not more than 105 per cent of the estimated potency unless otherwise stated in the individual monograph.

This degree of precision is the minimum acceptable for determining that the final product complies with the official requirements and may be inadequate for those deciding, for example, the potency which should be stated on the label or used as the basis for calculating the quantity of an antibiotic to be incorporated in a preparation. In such circumstances, assays of greater precision may be desirable with, for instance, fiducial limits of error of the order of 98 per cent to 102 per cent. With this degree of precision, the lower fiducial limit lies close to the estimated potency. By using this limit, instead of the estimated potency, to assign a potency to the antibiotic either for labelling or for calculating the quantity to be included in a preparation, there is less likelihood of the final preparation subsequently failing to comply with the official requirements for potency.

STERILITY TESTING OF PHARMACEUTICALS

39

Sterility Testing of Pharmaceuticals

According to Indian Pharmacopoeia (1996) the sterility testings are intended for detecting the presence of viable forms of microorganisms in or on Pharmacopoeia preparations. Sterility test critically assesses whether a sterilized pharmaceutical product is free from contaminating microorganisms or not. The main objective of this test is to ensure that the batch of the product is sterile or has been sterilized.

Sterility test is exclusively based on the principle that in case the bacteria are strategically placed in a specific medium that caters for the requisite nutritive material and water and maintained duly at a favorable temperature of $37 \pm 2°C$, the microorganisms have a tendency to grow and their legitimate presence may be clearly indicated by the appearance of a turbidity in the originally clear medium. However, very low levels of contamination cannot be detected on the basis of the random sampling of a batch. Moreover, if contamination is not uniform throughout the batch random sampling cannot detect contamination with certainty. Since every container cannot be tested, a significant number of containers should be examined to give a suitable degree of confidence in the results of the test. Table 1 gives the guidance on the minimum number of items in the batch on the assumption that the preparation has been manufactured under conditions designed to exclude contamination.

Table 1 Minimum number of items recommended to be tested in relation to the number of items in the batch.

Number of items in the batch	Minimum number of items recommended for testing.
1. Injectable preparations	
a. Not more than 100 containers	10% or 4 containers whichever is greater
b. More than 100 but not more than 500 containers	10 containers
c. More than 500 containers	2% or 20 containers whichever is less

Table 1 *Contd…*

Number of items in the batch	Minimum number of items recommended for testing.
2. Ophthalmic and other non-injectable preparations	
a. Not more than 200 containers	5% or 2 containers whichever is greater
b. More than 200 containers	10 containers
3. Surgical dressings	
Not more than 100 packages	
More than 100 but not more than 500 packages	1% or 4packages whichever os greater
More than 100 packages	10 packages
	2% or 20 packages whichever is less

Minimum number of products to be tested in each batch is given in table 2

Table 2 Minimum amount of product to be tested in medium

Contents in container	Minimum quantity of product	Minimum volume of culture medium (ml)
For Liquids:		
a. Less than 1ml	Total content	15
b. 1ml or more but less than 5ml	Half the content	20
c. 5ml or more but not less than 20ml	2ml	20
	5ml	80
d. 20ml or more but not less than 50ml	10ml	80
e. 50ml or more but less than 100ml		
For Solids:		
a. Less than 50mg	Total content	40
b. 50mg or more but less than 200mg	Half the content	80
	100mg	80
c. 20mg or more		

There are two methods of sterility testing

1. Direct inoculation

2. Membrane filtration

1. Direct inoculation method:

In direct inoculation method, transfer the quantity of the preparation to be examined as prescribed in table directly into culture medium so that the volume of the product is not more than 10% of the volume of the medium, unless otherwise prescribed. If the product is to be examined has antimicrobial activity, carry out the test after neutralizing this with a suitable neutralizing substance (polysorbate 80 at a concentration of 10g/l).

Requirements:

Fluid thioglycollate medium

Soyabean-casin digest medium

polysorbate 80

Method of test varies according to substance to be examined:

a. Aqueous solutions and suspensions

b. Oily liquids

c. Ointment and creams

d. solids

e. sterile devices

f. Transfusion or Infusion Assemblies

A. Aqueous solutions and suspensions:

The actual tests for microbial contamination are invariably performed on the same sample using recommended media. In certain cases when the amount present in a single container is quite insufficient to carry out the stipulated tests, the combined contents of either two or more containers may be employed to inoculate the above stated media.

Methodology:

1. Sample from the container must be removed carefully with a sterile pipette or with a sterile syringe.

2. Transfer aseptically, the prescribed volume of the substance from each container to a vessel of the culture medium.

3. Mix the liquid with the medium carefully taking care not to aerate excessively.

4. Incubate the inoculated media for not less than 14 days (unless otherwise mentioned) at 30-35°C for fluid thioglycollate medium and 20-25°C for soyabean-casein digest medium.

5. Maintain both negative and positive controls

Important points:

1. In case, the substance under investigation renders the culture medium turbid whereby the presence or absence of the actual microbial growth may not be determined conveniently and readily by sheer visual examination, it is always advisable and recommended that a suitable transfer of a certain portion of the medium to other fresh vessel of the same medium between the 3rd and 7th days after the said test actually commenced.

2. Subsequently, continue the incubation of the said transfer vessel for not less than 7 additional days after transfer, and for a total of not more than 14 days.

B. Oils and oily solutions:

For carrying out test for bacterial contamination of oils and oily solutions it is recommended to make use of culture media to which octylphenoxypolyethoxy ethanol has been added. However, these emulsifying agents should not exhibit any inherent antimicrobial characteristic features under prevailing parameters of the test.

The required test must be carried out as already described under aqueous solutions and suspensions

Important points:

1. Tests comprising of oily preparations should be shaken gently every day

2. When fluid thioglycollate medium is used for detection of the anaerobic microorganisms shaking or mixing must be restricted to a bare minimum level so as to maintain perfect anaerobic experimental parameters.

C. Ointments:

1. Carefully prepare the test sample by diluting 10 times in sterile diluents for instance fluid B or any other suitable aqueous vehicle which is capable of dispensing the test material homogeneously throughout the fluid mixture.

2. Mix 10ml of the fluid mixture thus obtained with 80ml of the medium and subsequently proceed as per the method given under aqueous solutions and suspensions.

D. Solids:

1. Transfer carefully the required amount of the preparation under examination to the quantity of culture medium as specified in the table and mix thoroughly.

2. Incubate the inoculated media for not less than 14 days, unless otherwise specified at 30-35°C in the particular instance of fluid thioglycollate medium and at 20-25°C in the specific cases of soyabean-casein digest medium.

E. Sterile devices:

For articles of such size and shape as allow the complete immersion is not more than 1L of the culture medium test the intact article, using the suitable media and incubating under Aqueous solutions and suspensions.

F. Transfusion and infusion assemblies:

For transfusion or infusion assemblies or where the size of an item almost renders immersion impracticable and exclusively the liquid pathway should be sterile by all means, flush carefully the lumen of each of twenty units with a sufficient quantum of fluid thioglycollate medium and the lumen of each of 20 units with a sufficient quantum of soyabean casein digest medium to give an ultimate recovery of not less than 15ml of each medium. Finally, incubate with not less than 100mL of each of the two media as prescribed under section Aqueous solutions and suspensions.

Exception: For such medical devices wherein the lumen is so small such that fluidthioglycollate medium will not pass through easily, appropriately substitute alternate thioglycollate medium instead of the usual fluid thioglycollate medium and incubate that duly inoculated medium anaerobically.

Note : In such situations where the presence of the specimen under examination, in the culture medium critically interferes with the test by virtue of the ensuing bacteriostatic or fungistatic action, rinse the article thoroughly with the bare minimum quantum of *fluid A*. Finally recover the rinsed fluid and carry out the 'test' as stated under 'Membrane Filtration' for Sterile Devices.

Observation and Interpretation of Results:

In the case of direct inoculation, the various observation and interpretation of results may be accomplished by taking into consideration the following cardinal factors, such as:

1. Both at intervals during the incubation period, and at its completion, the media may be examined thoroughly for the critical macroscopic evidence of the bacterial growth.

2. In the event of a negative evidence, the 'sample' under examination passes the 'tests for sterility'.

3. If positive evidence of microbial growth is found, reserve the containers exhibiting this, and unless it is amply proved and adequately demonstrated by any other means that their (microorganisms) presence is on account such causes unrelated to the 'sample' being examined ; and, therefore, the tests for sterility are pronounced invalid. In such cases, it may be recommended to carry out a 'retest' employing an identical number of samples and volumes to be tested, and the media as in the original test.

4. Even then, if no evidence of microbial growth is duly observed, the 'sample' under investigation precisely passes the 'tests for sterility'.

5. In case, reasonable evidence of bacterial growth is observed, one may go ahead with the isolation and subsequent identification of the organisms.

6. If they are found to be not readily distinguishable from those (microbes) growing in the containers reserved for the very First Test, the 'sample' under investigation fails the 'tests for sterility'.

7. In case, the microorganisms are readily distinguishable from the ones actually growing in the containers reserved in the 'First Test', it is very much advisable to carry out a 'Second Retest' by employing virtually twice the number of samples.

8. Importantly, if no evidence of bacterial growth is observed in the 'Second Retest', the sample under examination legitimately passes the 'tests for sterility'.

9. Contrarily, if evidence of the growth of any microorganisms is duly observed in the 'second retest', the sample under investigation obviously fails the 'tests for sterility'.

2. Membrane filtration method:

This method is employed where substances to be examined is an oil, an ointment, a non-bacteriostatic solid not readily soluble in culture medium and a soluble powder or a liquid consisting of bacteriostatic or fungistatic properties.

The sample under investigation is carefully filtered via a hydrophobic-edged membrane filter that would precisely retain any possible contaminating microorganisms. The resulting membrane is duly washed in situ to get rid of any possible 'traces of antibiotic' that would have been sticking to the surface of the membrane intimately. Finally, the segregated microorganisms are meticulously transferred to the suitable culture media under perfect aseptic environment.

Requirements:

Fluid thioglycollate medium (to test for aerobic and anaerobic bacteria)

Soyabean-casein digest medium (for fungi and aerobic bacteria)

NaOH (1N)

Test tubes

Millipore membrane (0.45)

Membrane filtration assembly

A. Diluent fluid A: Dissolve 1g peptic digest of animal tissue eg. Bacteriological peptone or its equivalent in water to make up the volume up to 1L, filter or centrifuge to clarify, and adjust to pH 7.1±0.2, dispense 100ml into flasks and sterilize in an autoclave at 121°C for 20 minutes.

Note: In a specific instance, where Fluid A is to be used in carrying out the tests for sterility on a specimen of the penicillin or cephalosporin class of antibiotics, aseptically incorporate an amount of sterile penicillinase enzyme to the Fluid A to be employed to rinse the membrane(s) sufficient to inactivate any residual antibiotic activity on the membrane(s) after the solution of the specimen has been duly filtered.

B. Diluent fluid B: when the test sample contains lecithin or oil add 1ml of polysorbate 80/litre of diluent, adjust pH t0 7.1 ± 0.2, dispense into flasks and sterilize at 121°C for 20 minutes.

Note: A sterile fluid shall not have either antimicrobial or antifungal properties if it is to be considered suitable for dissolving, diluting or rinsing a preparation being examined for sterility.

Methodology:

1. Clean the outer surface of vials, bottles, ampoules with 70% Isopropyl alcohol or ethanol and keep in aseptic condition. However, if the contents are packed in the container packed under vacuum, introduce sterile air through a needle attached to a syringe barrel filled with nonabsorbent cotton in aseptic condition.

2. Take the quantity of the sample to be tested as prescribed in table

3. Assemble the sterile filtration unit and placing a sterile Millipore filter (0.45μ) into the holder of equal diameter.

4. A small quantity of fluid A is transferred on the membrane to moist the membrane filter.

5. Aseptically open the seal of vial(s) as prescribed in table, draw liquid with sterile pipette or syringe and filter through membrane filter (if sample is filtrate solid, dissolve into sterile diluent and use as liquid) however, if the liquid sample has antibiotic properties, wash the membrane filter three times with 100ml fluid A each time).

6. After filtration, aseptically remove the membrane from the holder of the unit and cut the filter into two equal halves with sterile scissors.

7. Immerse one half of the membrane in 100ml of soyabean-casein digest medium and incubate at 20-25°C for 7 days and the other half of the membrane in 100ml of fluid thioglycollate medium in tubes and incubate at 30-35°C for 7 days.

8. Maintain one negative and positive control along with the sample test tube.

Observation and Results:

1. If no growth is observed, in negative control and the test sample tube, it means the sample meets the requirements of sterility.

2. If microbial growth is seen in test sample tube and negative control, the experiment should be repeated as the place where the experiment was conducted was not in aseptic condition.

3. If the microbial growth is observed in test sample tube and no growth is seen in negative control tube that means the sample does not meet the requirement of sterility. The test should be repeated unless the same microorganism is observed.

*In all the cases growth should be seen in positive control tubes.

Precautions:

1. The tests for sterility must be carried out under highly aseptic conditions like laminar air flow so as to avoid any least possible accidental contamination of the product being examined.

2. The environment where the test for sterility is conducted must always be monitored at a definite periodical interval by environmental monitoring by plate exposure or by sampling of air.

3. Maintaining suitable positive and negative controls is must in sterility test.

Fluid thioglycollate medium

(to test for aerobic and anaerobic bacteria)

L-cystine	0.5g
NaCl	2.5g
Dextrose	5.5g
Granular agar	0.75g

Yeast extract	5.0g
Pancreatic digest of casein	15.0g
Sodium thioglycollate	0.5g
or thioglycollic acid	0.3ml
Resazurin (1.1% fresh solution)	1.0ml
Distilled water	1L
pH	7.1±0.2

Soybean casein-digest agar medium

(for fungi and aerobic bacteria)

Pancreatic digest of casein	17.0g
Papain digest of soyabean meal	3.0g
NaC	5.0g
Dibasic potassium phosphate	2.5g
Dextrose	2.5g
Distilled water	1L
pH	7.1±0.2

ENVIRONMENTAL MONITORING

40

Environmental Monitoring by Settling Plate Method

Environmental monitoring is an inspection of the working environment in different locations of the plant for airborne microorganisms which may contaminate or affect industrial products. Microbiological monitoring is a surveillance system for microbiological control which provides monitoring, testing and feedback to the microbiology quality levels in aseptic environments. Air monitoring is therefore particularly important where pharmaceutical products are manufactured in clean room areas with filtered air. Settle plates are useful for qualitative analysis of airborne microorganisms and for revealing trends in airborne contamination. Settling plate enables continuous and efficient monitoring of micro-organisms during production processes. Viable biological particles sediment out of the air and settle onto the plate's surface over the time of exposure.

Materials required:

Petri plates

Nutrient agar medium (or)

Soyabean Casein Digest Agar medium

Procedure:

1.   Prepare nutrient agar or soyabean casein digest agar medium and sterilize in autoclave at 121°C for 15 minutes.

2.   When medium is cooled to 45°C pour into sterile Petri plates and allowed to solidify so as to form uniform layer.

3.   Incubate the prepared plates for 24 hrs in incubator at 37°C to check for any contamination or improper autoclaving.

4.   If no growth is seen, label the place of exposure and date on all the plates using glass marker.

5. Later open the lid completely and expose the plates at different areas of microbiology laboratory, outside the lab and inside laminar air flow for about 4 hours.

6. At the end of exposure time, collect all the plates by replacing the lids of respective plates and incubate at 37°C for 24-48 hrs by inverting the plates.

7. At the end of incubation period observe the number of bacterial colonies on agar surface of Petri plates of different locations and make a note using colony counter and compare the microbial count of each location.

8. Now place all the Petri plates in incubator at 25°C for 5 days.

9. At the end of incubation observe the plates for fungal colonies and make a note and compare the colonies at each location.

Observation table

S.No.	Place of exposure	No of bacterial colonies	No of fungal colonies
1.	At the entrance of the lab		
2.	At corner of the lab		
3.	Center of the lab		
4.	LAF		
5	Outside the lab		

Precautions:

1. Use always two days preincubated plates

2. Before exposing check the plates for any microbial contamination

3. Expose and collect the plates in such a away to avoid personal interference

4. Open the lid of plate in such a way that fingers does not touch surface of the medium

5. Sterilize the exposed plates in autoclave before discarding the medium

Nutrient agar medium

Peptone	5.0g
Beef extract	3.0g
NaCl	5.0g
Agar	15.0g
Distilled water-	1000mL

Soyabean Casein Digest Agar medium:

Pancreatic digest of Casein	15g
Papain digest of soyabean	5g
Sodium chloride	5g
Agar	15g
pH	7.3
Distilled water	1000mL

BACTERIAL ANALYSIS OF WATER

41

Bacterial Examination of Water by Multiple Tube Fermentation Test

The bacterial examination of water is performed routinely by water utilities and many governmental agencies to ensure a safe supply of water. The examination is intended to identify water sources which have been contaminated by fecal matter, a series of tests are used to demonstrate the presence or absence of coliforms which are Gram negative, aerobic or facultative anaerobic, non endospore forming rods, capable of fermenting lactose with the production of acid and gas within 24 hours of incubation at 37°C. Two organisms in this group include *Escherichia coli* and *Enterobacter aerogenes*. However, the only true fecal coli form is *E.coli* which is found only in the fecal matter of warm blooded animals. The presence of this organism in a water supply is evidence of recent fecal contamination. Coliform bacteria in a given water sample is estimated by multiple tube fermentation test which are indicators of fecal contamination. The estimation of coliforms is carried out sequentially in three stages

a. Presumptive

b. Confirmed

c. Completed test

A. Presumptive test:

The test is used to detect and estimate coliform bacterial population in a water sample. The test is known as presumptive because of the development of a positive result in Mac Conkey broth inoculated with water. In this test known volume of test sample water is added to lactose fermentation tubes and production of acid and gas from the fermentation of lactose is a positive test for the coliform bacteria. The presence of acid is indicated by colour change of the medium and production of gas is detected as gas bubble collected in the inverted Durhams tube inserted in the medium. A statistical method is used to estimate the presence of population of coliform expressed as the most probable number (MPN). A count of number of lactose fermentation tubes showing production of gas following incubation period is taken and MPN is found by matching the results with those provided in the statistical table.

Requirements:

1. Water sample
2. 9ml single strength lactose fermentation broth tubes (6 no),
3. 10ml double strength lactose fermentation broth tubes (3 no),
4. Sterile pipettes (one each of 10ml, 1ml and 0.1ml).
5. Mac Conkey broth or lactose broth
6. Eosin methylene blue (EMB) agar
7. Test tubes of 5ml,10ml,20ml
8. Durham's tubes
9. Nutrient agar slants
10. Incubator
11. Laminar air flow
12. Sterile pipettes
13. Glass marker
14. Gram staining kit

Procedure:

1. Collect the water sample in a sterile glass bottle or conical flasks.
2. Lable 3 single strength lactose broth tubes or Mac Conkey broth tubes as 0.1, another 3 tubes as 1.0 and 3 double strength broth tubes as 10.
3. Insert all the tubes with Durhams tube.
4. Inoculate aseptically 0.1 tubes with 0.1 sample with the help of 0.1 ml sterile pipette.
5. Inoculate aseptically 1labelled tubes with 1ml sample using 1.0ml sterile pipette.
6. Inoculate aseptically 10 labelled tubes with 10ml sample using 10ml sterile pipette.

7. Incubate all the 9 tubes at 37°C for 24 hours. Observe for production of acid and gas.

8. Read the MPN index/100 ml from a standard table.

Note: If presumptive test is negative, no further testing is performed and water is considered to be microbiologically safe.

B. Confirmed coliform test:

This test is used to confirm the presence of coliforms in water sample showing positive or doubtful presumptive test. In the confirmed test, the samples from the positive presumptive lactose broth are streaked on to a selective differential medium for coliforms. The medium commonly used is eosin methylene blue (EMB) agar which is a selective medium as methylene blue inhibits the growth of gram (+) ve bacteria. The medium is also differential as it gives colored colonies of lactose fermenting bacteria due to the formation of a complex. Non-lactose fermenters produce colorless colonies on EMB agar.

Requirements:

Lactose broth culture from presumptive test

Eosin methylene blue agar plates

Laminar air flow

Inoculation loop

Procedure:

1. Streak EMB agar plates with 24 hour lactose broth tubes showing test positive with a sterile inoculating loop.

2. Incubate the plates for 24-48 hours at 37°C in an inverted position.

3. Examine the inoculated plate for the presence or absence of *E.coli* colonies.

Observation and results: Appearance of typical coliform colonies (*E.coli*) with dark centres and metallic sheen is a confirmed test for the presence of coliforms and indicates that the water is non-potable.

C. Completed coliform test:

The completed test is used as a further confirmatory test for the presence of *E.coli* in water sample. In this test lactose positive colonies from EMB agar are isolated and inoculated into a lactose broth tube and streaked on a nutrient agar plate with the help of inoculation loop. Acid and gas production in lactose broth, confirms the presence of *E.coli* in a given sample.

Requirements:

1. 24 hour incubated EMB agar plates of Confirmed test
2. Lactose fermentation broth tubes,
3. Nutrient agar slants and gram stain kit.

Procedure:

1. Inoculate fermentation broth tubes with isolated coliform colonies of EMB agar plates using inoculating loop and insert a Durhams tube for detection of gas.
2. Streak nutrient agar slant with colony from EMB agar plate using inoculating loop.
3. Incubate the inoculated broth tubes and slants at 37°C for 24hours
4. Stain the bacteria with the help of Gram stain.

Observation and results:

Examine the lactose fermentation broth tubes for the production of acid and gas. Observe the slides for Gram reaction. Production of acid and gas in the fermentation tubes and Gram –ve rods on the slides confirms the presence of coliforms.

Table: Most probable number (MPN) of coliform bacteria present in 100ml ater for various combinations of positive and negative results when three each of 10ml, 1ml and three 0.1ml sample portions are used

Number of tubes giving positive reactions

3 of 10 ml	3 of 1 ml	3 of 0.1 ml	MPN Inded
0	0	1	3
0	1	0	3
1	0	0	4
1	0	1	7
1	1	1	11
1	2	0	11
2	0	0	9
2	0	1	14
2	1	0	15
2	1	1	20
2	2	0	21
3	0	0	23
3	0	1	39
3	0	2	64
3	1	0	43
3	1	1	75
3	1	2	120
3	2	0	93
3	2	1	150
3	2	2	210
3	3	0	240
3	3	1	460
3	3	1	1100
3	3	3	2400

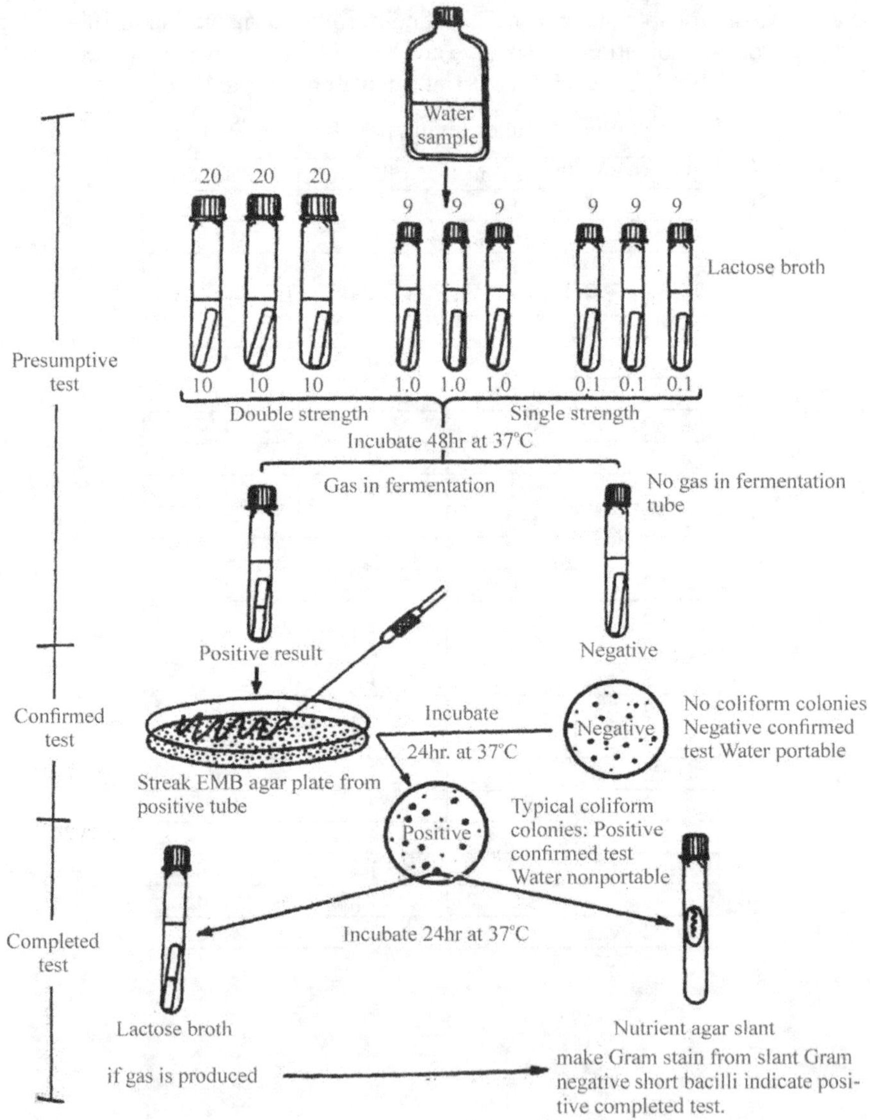

Standard procedure for bacterial analysis of water

Media composition:

Mac Conkey's broth

Bacto peptone	17.0g
Proteose peptone	3.0
Lactose	10.0g
Bile salts mixture	1.5g
NaCl	5.0g
Neutral red	0.03g
Crystal violet	0.001g

1. **Eosin methylene blue (EMB) agar**

Peptone	10g
Lactose	10g
K_2HPO_4	2.0g
Eosin Y	0.4g
Methylene blue	0.065g
Agar	15g
Distilled water	1L
pH	7.1

2. **Lactose medium**

Beef extract	3.0g
Peptone	5.0g
Lactose	5.0g
Water	1L

For double strength use twice the concentration of the ingredients

42

Bacteriological Examination of Water by Membrane Filtration Method

In this method water sample to be tested is passed through membrane filters capable of retaining microorganisms larger than 0.45 μm. The membrane filter containing bacteria is placed on agar medium and incubated for 24 hours. The developed colonies are counted. This method offers several advantages over the conventional multiple tube method of water analysis, results are available in the shorter period of time, and the results are readily reproducible because of high accuracy.

Requirements:

Water sample

Membrane filtration unit

Endo MF agar

Sterile membrane filter

Suction pump

Foreceps

Procedure:

1. Prepare endo MF agar medium and distribute into Petri plates

2. Assemble the sterilized filtration unit and aseptically place a sterile membrane filter on the holder of the filtration unit.

3. Attach the side arm of the flask with a vacuum pump through a rubber pipe and pour the measured quantity of water in the funnel fitted to the filtration unit. Generally, 50ml water is used for filtration.

4. Switch on the vacuum pump and the entire sample will be filtered, wash the inner surface of the funnel with 20 ml of sterile water.

5.   Disconnect the vacuum, unclamp the filter assembly and remove the membrane filter with a sterile forceps and place it on the prepared agar plates and incubate at 37°C for 24 hours and calculate the number of colonies per ml of sample.

Observation and results:

At the end of incubation period count the number of colonies in two plates and take the average of two plates.

Note: Follow aseptic technique throughout the procedure

Multiple fermentation tube technique	Membrane filter technique
Slower: requires 48 hours for a positive	More rapid: quantitative results in or presumptive positive about 18 hours
More labour-intensive	Less labour-intensive
Requires more culture medium	Requires less culture medium
Requires more glassware	Requires less glassware
More sensitive	Less sensitive
Result obtained indirectly by statistical approximation (low precision)	Results obtained directly by colony count (high precision)
Not readily adaptable for use in the field	Readily adapted for use in the field
Applicable to all types of water	Not applicable to turbid waters
Consumables readily available in most countries	Cost of consumables is high in many countries
May give better recovery of stressed or damaged organisms in some circumstances	

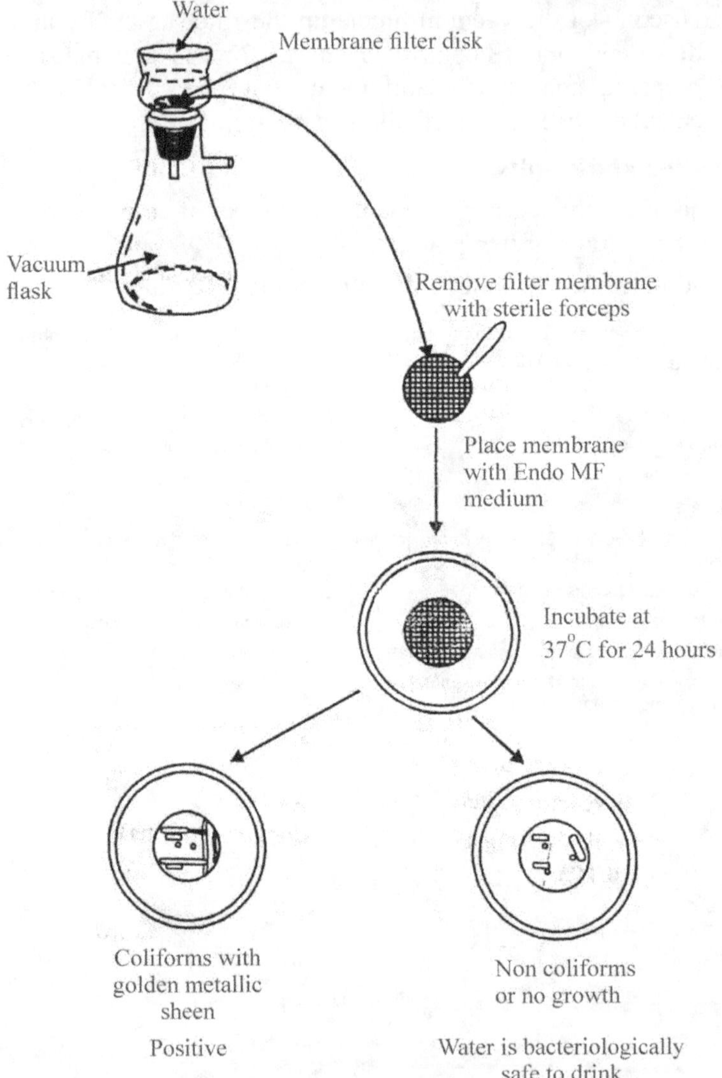

Process of coliforms detection by membrane filtration technique

43

Analysis of Water for Total Bacterial Population by Standard Plate Count

In this method, the sample to be tested is plated in the agar plate and bacteria are allowed to grow and the colonies thus developed are counted. This method can also be used for plate count of milk, dairy products etc. For accurate analysis, it is recommended to plate the samples in duplicate and take the average.

Requirements:

Tryptone glucose extract agar

Water samples/milk samples

Petri dishes

Laminar air flow

Sterile pipettes

Procedure:

1. Collect water sample in a sterile glass bottle.
2. Prepare tryptone glucose extract agar media and distribute 20ml in tubes.
3. Sterilize the agar media tubes in the autoclave at 121°C for 15 minutes.
4. Transfer 1ml of water sample to each sterile Petri plates and pour media when cooled to 45° C.
5. After solidification of media, incubate the plates at 35°C for 24 hours.

Observation and results:

Bacterial colonies appeared on the surface of the plates are counted and the average of two plates is recorded.

Important points

1. Depending upon the quality of water sample serial dilutions are performed and the bacterial count is multiplied by the dilution factor.

Tryptone glucose extract agar

Tryptone	20.0g
Glucose	5.0g
KH_2PO_4	0.20g
K_2HPO_4	0.35g
$MgCl_2.6H_2O$	0.10g
$CaCl_2.2H_2O$	0.07g
Agar	15g
Distilled water	1L

MICROBIAL TAXONOMY

44

Fungi

Fungi are a diverse group of eukaryotic organisms that occupy a variety of habitats. They are neither a plant nor an animal. They are devoid of chlorophil and obtain nutrients by absorbtion. Fungi live as parasites (which feed on a living host causing it harm) or saprophytes (feed on dead and decaying organic matter by producing a range of hydrolytic enzymes). Some are facultative parasites of plants and animals and some form symbiotic relation with other organisms. Majority of fungal species are composed of filamentous hyphae and are often referred to as moulds, whereas the yeast are unicellular fungi. The basic unit of a fungus is hyphae which is a thread like structure having a cell wall made up of chitin and ergosterol. Hypha grows out of germinating spores. A net work of hyphae is called mycelium. Fungi are of both beneficial and harmful. Beneficial fungi are helpful in decaying dead material and are important in recycling of nutrients, useful in producing antibiotics and in fermentation production of commercially important products. Harmful fungi cause disease in plants and animals, spoil food and spoil leather articles. Generally moulds reproduce by producing spores where as yeast reproduce by budding. Study of fungi is called mycology.

Features of some of the selected fungi
1. *Aspergillus*

Kingdom: Fungi
Division: Ascomycota
Class: Eurotiomycetes
Order: Eurotiales
Family: Trichochomaceae
Genus: Aspergillus

1. The Genus *Aspergillus* consists of mould species found in various habitats.
2. Colonies are usually fast growing and are of various colours. Initially white then turn to yellow, yellow-brown, green-brown to black or shades of green.
3. Vegetative mycelium septate,branched, hyphae colourless.
4. Conidia develop as stalk heads from footcell producing conidiophores at long axis.
5. Conidiophores septate or unseptate broadening into elliptical, hemispherical or globose fertile vesicles.
6. Vesicles bear phialides in one series or two series.
7. Phialides cluster in terminal groups or radiating from entire surface
8. Conidia elliptical, globose, smoothwalled, rough or spinulose walls produced in chains.
9. Some species of *Aspergillus* have commercial applications.
10. The diseases caused by few species of *Aspergillus* is called Aspergillosis.

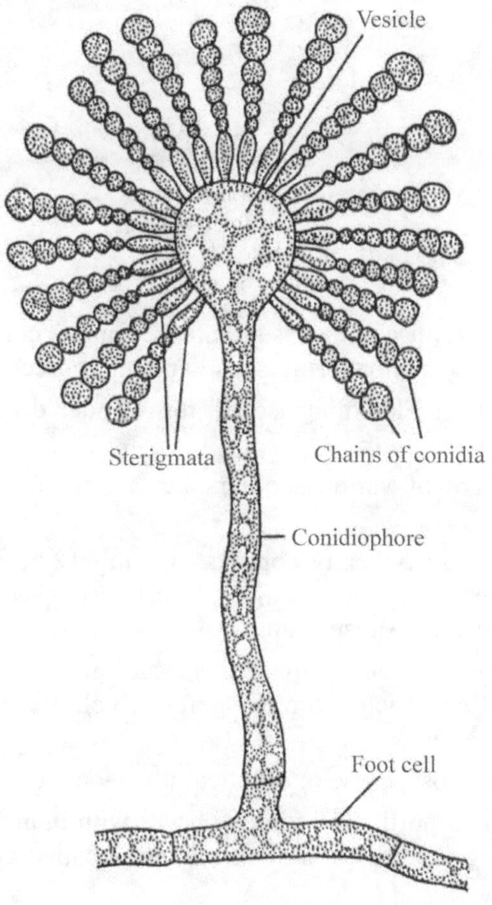

Aspergillus

2. *Penicillium*

Kingdom: Fungi
Division: Ascomycota
Class: Eurotiomycetes
Order: Eurotiales
Family: Trichochomaceae
Genus: Penicillium

1. *Penicillium* is a common saprophytic fungus commonly found on decaying organic matter. It is also known as green or blue mould.

2. Sir Alexander Flemming isolatd the wonder drug, penicillin from *Penicillium notatum*.

3. Colonies are of various colours i.e. green, bluish green, greyish green.

4. The mycelium typically consists of a highly branched network of multinucleate, septate, usually colourless hyphae which run in all directions on the substratum.

5. Many branched conidiophores sprout on the mycelium bearing individual constricted conidiospores which are the main dispersal route of the fungi.

6. Conidia globose, ovate or elliptical ith smooth or rough surface.

7. The terminal portion of conidiophores with branches and chains of conidia together looks like broom and is called penicillus-meaning broom.

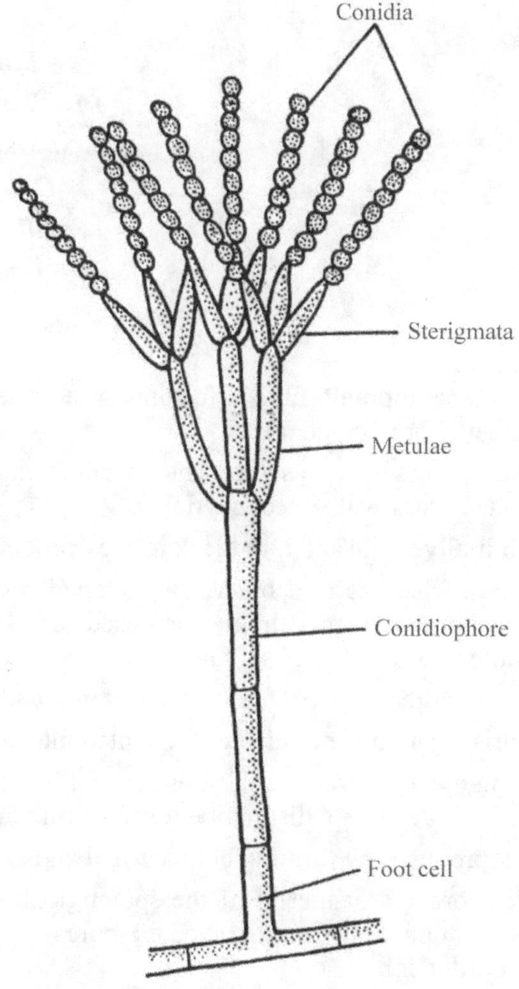

Penicillium

3. *Rhizopus*

Kingdom: *Fungi*
Division: *Zygomycota*
Class: *Mucoromycotina*
Order: *Mucorales*
Family: *Mucoraceae*
Genus: *Rhizopus*

1. *Rhizopus* is a saprophytic fungus feeding on a variety of organic matter, parasitic or pathogenic.
2. The fungal species grow as filamentous branching hyphae that generally lack cross-walls (ceonocytic).
3. Colonies initially white and turn black as they produce spores.
4. The fungus is characterised by well developed, richly branched and rapidly growing mycelium composed of three types of hyphae: stolons, rhizoids and sporangiophores.
5. The stolons are present at place to place forming nodes.
6. Rhizoids arise from nodes and later implanted into substratum.
7. The sporangiophores arise aerially either singly or in groups of two, three or more among distinctive root like rhizoids.
8. *Rhizopus* reproduces by forming both asexual and sxual spores.
9. The black sporangia at the tip of the sporangiophores are round and produce numerous multinucleate spores at maturity for asexual reporduction.
10. *Rhizopus* reproduces sexually when two compatible and physiologically distinct mycelia are present forming a dark zygospore at the point where two compatible mycelia fuse.Upon germination, a zygospore produces colonies.
11. *Rhizopus* spp. Are among the fungi causing group of infections called as Zygomycosis.
12. Many members of the Rhizopus have commercial industrial applications.

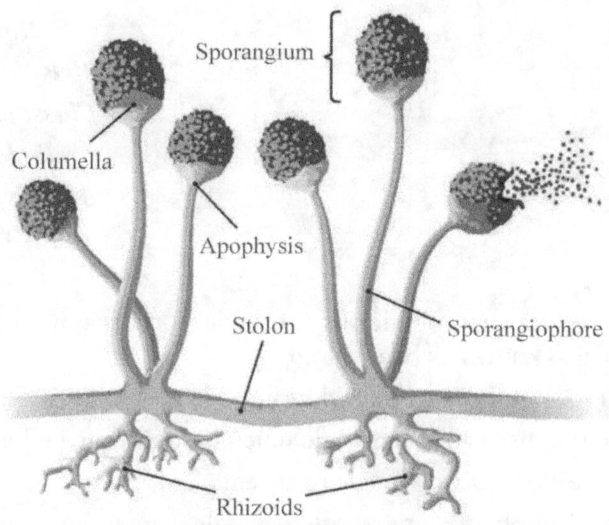

Structure of Rhizopus

4. *Mucor*

Kingdom: Fungi
Division: Zygomycota
Class: Mucomycotina
Order: Mucorales
Family: Mucoraceae
Genus: Mucor

1. *Mucor* is a saprophytic fungi growing on decaying organic matter. It is also known as black mold.
2. Colonies initially white and turn to black at maturity.
3. *Mucor* consists of coenocytic much branched mycelium.
4. Unlike *Rhizopus* rhizoids are absent.
5. Sporangiophores are shorter, single, emerging from mycelium forming a thick tuft, erect, unbranched with terminal sporangia.
6. Sporangiophore is extended to form columella which protrudes in to sporangium.
7. Spores are released by rupture of sporangium which germinates to form a new mycelium on substratum.
8. Compatable strains form short specialized hyphae called gametangia during sexual reproduction and fuse to form a thick walled spherical zygosporangium which contains zygospore.

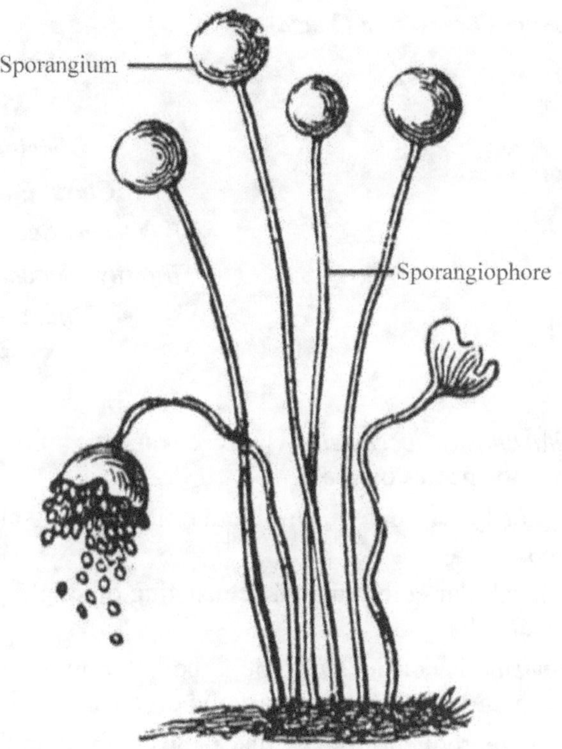

Structure of Mucor

5. *Saccharomyces cerevisiae (Yeast)*

Kingdom: Fungi
Division: Ascomycota
Class: Saccharomycetes
Order: Saccharomycetales
Family: Saccharomycetaceae
Genus: Saccharomyces
Species: cerevisiae

1. *Saccharomyces cerevisiae* is a eukaryotic unicellular fungus belongs to species of yeast.

2. It is mostly saprophyte and found in sugary substrates (sugar fungus).

3. It is unicellular edible fungus, consisting of single minute, oval or spherical cell.

4. *S.cerevisiae* is considered to be a model organism by scientists as it is both a uniellular and eukaryotic organism.

5. Asexual reproduction takes place mostly by budding and binary fission. Sexual reproduction takes place by plasmogamy, karyogamy and meiosis.

6. The cells secrete enzymes on the substratum which are collectively called zymase. The enzyme changes starch or complex sugars into simple sugars.

7. *S.cerevisiae* is famously known for its role in food production. It is the critical component in the fermentation process that converts sugar into alcohol; an ingredient shared in beer, wine and distilled beverages.

8. It is also used in the baking process as a leaving agent; yeast releasing gas into their environment results in the spongy like texture of breads and cakes.

9. *S.cerevisiae* is commonly called brewer's yeast, bakers yeast, as well as wine yeast and distiller's yeast.

10. It is commercially used in industry for the production of ethylalcohol on large scale.

11. Compressed yeast is used as the source of vitamins. While fresh yeast cells are excellent source of single cell protein (SCP) and vitamin B complex.

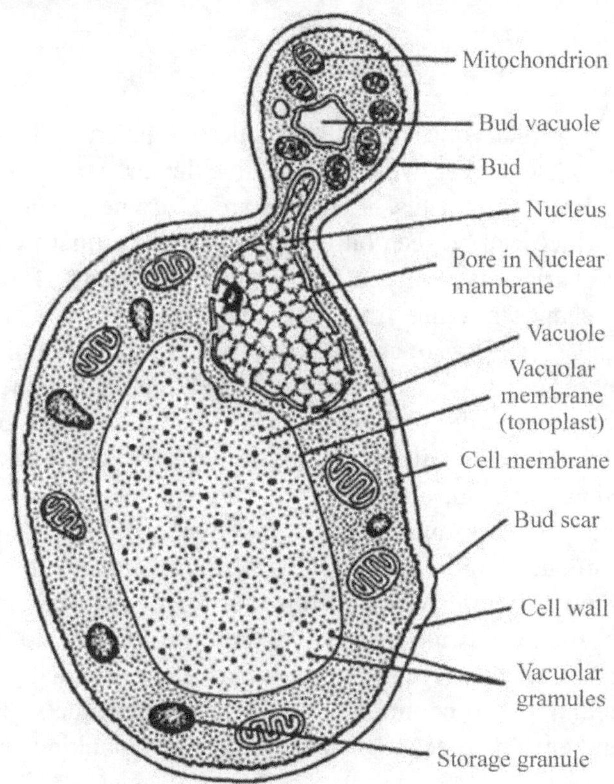

Budding cell of *Saccharomyces cerevisiae*

45

Bacteria

Bacteria are prokaryotic unicellular microorganisms. They are omni present i.e. present everywhere. They live in air, water, soil, dust and bodies of other organisms. Bacteria are extremely small unicellular organisms which can be seen only with the aid of a microscope. The size of bacteria varies, typically a micrometre in length. Bacteria are of number of shapes ranging from cocci to rods and spirals. Though the shapes of most bacteria are constant, few can exist in several shapes, such a phenomenon is known as pleomorphism. Bacteria may be motile with flagella or non motile without flagella. They can be autotrophic or heterotrophic like parasitic, saprophytic or symbiotic. They carry out asexual (Binary fission, endospore) and sexual methods of reproduction (Transformation, transduction and conjugation). Based on staining, bacteria can be Gram negative with more lipid content and less peptidoglycon or Gram positive with more peptidoglycon and less lipid content in their cellwall. Many bacteria are useful to mankind by increasing soil fertility, recycling of nutrients, in producing a number of antibiotics and other commercially applicable products. Few bacteria cause a number of diseases to plants, animals and mankind and cause a lot of damage.

1. *Actinomycetes*

Domain*: Bacteria*
Phylum*: Actinobacteria*
Class*: Actinobactria*
Subclass*: Actinobacteridae*
Order*: Actinomycetales*

1. Actinomycetes are a group of Gram-positive, spore forming, aerobic bacteria. Morphologically they resemble fungi because of their elongated cells that branch into filaments or hyphae. These are the organisms with characteristics common to both bacteria and fungi.

2. Actinomycetes are numerous and widely distributed in soil, compost etc.

3. They degrade recalcitrant compounds like chitin and cellulose.

4. The actinomycetes group includes bacteria like *Mycobacterium* (the causal agent of tuberculosis and leprosy), *Corynebacterium* (a common commensal on human skin) and *Streptomyces* (the source of many antibiotics as well as the epleasant odor of freshly turned soil).

5. The common genera of Actinomycetes abundently found in soil are *Streptomyces, Nocardia* and *Micromonospora*.

6. Few species are pathogenic to humans.

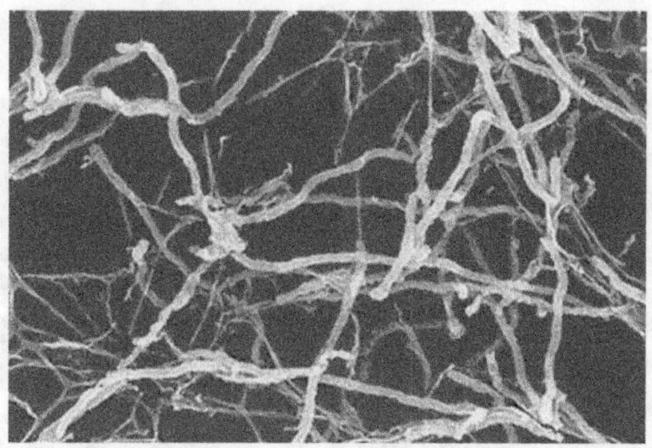

Structure of *Actinomycetes*

2. *Bacillus*

Domain: *Bacteria*
Phylum: *Firmicutes*
Class: *Bacilli*
Order: *Bacillales*
Family: *Bacillaceae*
Genus: *Bacillus*

1. The genus *Bacillus* is Gram positive, rod shaped, motile, endospore-forming bacteria.

2. They occur in wide range of habitats and few are pathogenic.

3. *Bacillus* species may be obligate aerobes or facultative anaerobes, usually catalase positive.

4. Under unfavourable conditions members of genus *Bacillus* produce endospores which remain dormant for very long periods.

5. Many *Bacillus* species are capable of producing enzymes like proteases, amylases lipases and other commercially important products.

6. Some of the examples of *Bacillus* species are *Bacillus subtilis*, *B.licheniformis*, *B.amyloliquifaciens*, *B.cereus*, *B.megaterium*, *B.polymyxa*, *B.pumilus* etc.

7. *Bacillus subtilis* is one of the best understood prokaryotes and used as model organism.

8. Medically significant *Bacillus* species are *B.anthrax*, which causes anthrax and *B.cereus*, which causes food poisoning.

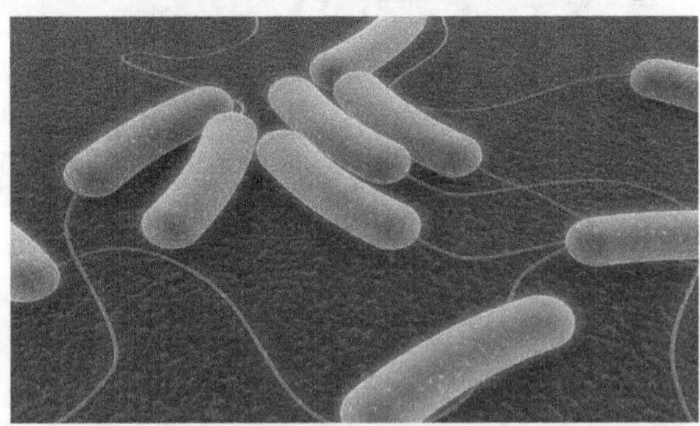

Structure of *Bacillus*

3. *Escherichia coli*

Domain: *Bacteria*
Phylum: *Proteobacteria*
Class: *Gammaproteobacteria*
Order: *Enterobacteriales*
Family: *Enterobacteriace*
Genus: *Escherichia*
Species: *coli*

1. *E.coli* is a Gram negative, facultative anaerobic, motile short rod, of the genus *Escherichia*.

2. It takes 20 minutes to reproduce under favourable conditions.

3. This bacterium is oxidase, catalase, methyl red and Voges Proskauer tests positive.

4. *E.coli* is generally found in the lower intestine of warm blooded organisms and expelled into the environment within fecal matter.

5. Most *E.coli* bacteria are harm less but few cause food poisoning by producing enterotoxin leading to diarrhoea.

6. Some bacteria form part of normal microbial flora of the gut and can benefit their hosts by producing vitamins and prevent colonization of the intestine with pathogenic bacteria, having symbiotic relation ship.

7. *E.coli* is the most widely studied prokaryotic model organism and most important species in biotechnology and microbiology fields.

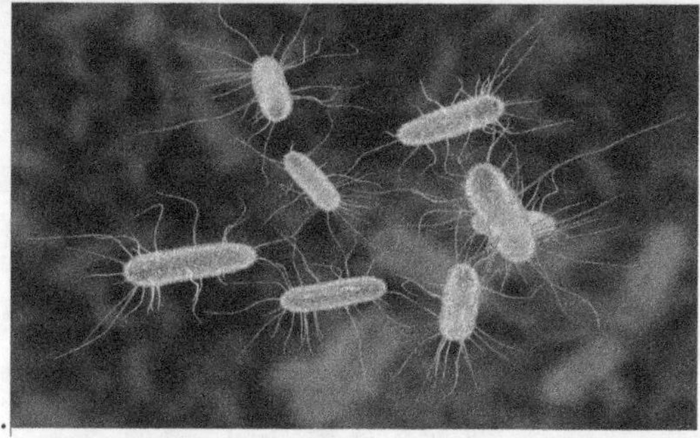

Structure of *Escherichia coli*

4. *Lactobaccillus*

Domain: Bacteria
Phylum: Firmicutes
Class: Bacilli
Order: Lactobacillales
Family: Lactobacillaceae
Genus: Lactobacillus

1. *Lactobacilli* are Gram positive, non-spore forming, rod shaped bacteria.

2. They are facultatively anaerobic, some times microaerophilic in nature.

3. *Lactobacilli* are nitrate reduction, glatin liquification and catalase and cytochrome tests negative.

4. These bacteria convert sugars to lactic acid forming major part of lactic acid bacteria group.

5. *Lactobacilli* form part of normal microbial flora at a number of body sites, such as the digestive system, urinary system and genital system and help in treating diarrhea, vaginal infections, digestion problems, colon inflammation and skin disorders etc.

6. These bacteria are the most common probiotic found in dairy products.

7. Some *Lactobacillus* species are used for commercial production of dairy products.

8. Some species have been associated with cases of dental caries (cavities).

9. Some of the examples of *Lactobacillus* species are *L.acidophilus, L.lactis, L.brevis, L.casei, L.plantarum* etc.

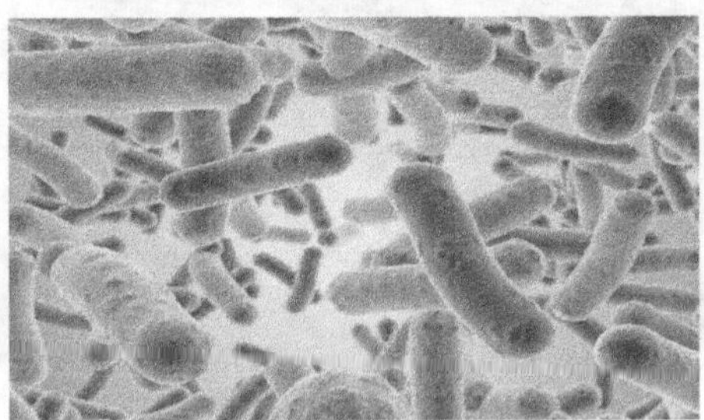

Structure of *Lactobacillus*

5. *Pseudomonas*

Domain*: Bacteria*
Phylum*: Proteobacteria*
Class*: Gammaproteobacteria*
Order*: Pseudomonadales*
Family*: Pseudomonadaceae*
Genus*: Pseudomonas*

1. These bacteria are aerobic, Gram-negative, motile rod shaped bacteria, known for their metabolic diversity.

2. These bacteria can be found in soil, water, plant and animal tissues. Many species are oppertunistic pathogens that affect humans, animals and plants.

3. *Pseudomonades* are common pathogens involved in infections acquired in hospital.

4. More than half of the clinical isolates produce pyocyanin, a blue-green pigment.

5. Healthy people are usually at low risk compared to patients with compromised host defence mechanisms.

6. Some of the examples of species of *Pseudomonas* are *P.aeruginosa, P.putida, P.alcaligenes, P.fluorescens etc.*

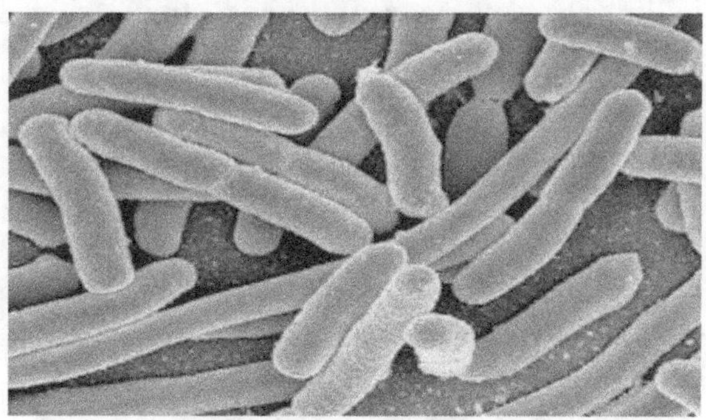

Structure of *Pseudomonas*

6. *Staphylococcus*

Domain: Bacteria
Phylum: Firmicutes
Class: Bacilli
Order: Bacillales
Family: Staphylococcaceae
Genus: Staphylococcus

1. *Staphylococci* are Gram positive, non-spore forming, non-motile, facultatively anaerobic spherical shaped bacteria.

2. These bacteria form grape-like clusters.

3. These bacteria are present in great numbers on the mucous membrane and skin, nose of humans and other warm-blooded animals and cause a variety of infections.

4. *Staphylococcus* usually infects immunocompromised humans and is an extremely versatile pathogen.

5. *S. aureus* is one of the major cause of hospital-acquired infection. It is responsible for mild skin and wound infections, invasive diseases and toxin mediated diseases etc.

6. *S.epidermidis* is a mild pathogen, opportunistic only in immuno compramised patients.

7. Methicillin-resistant *S.aureus* is one strain of great concern to humans.

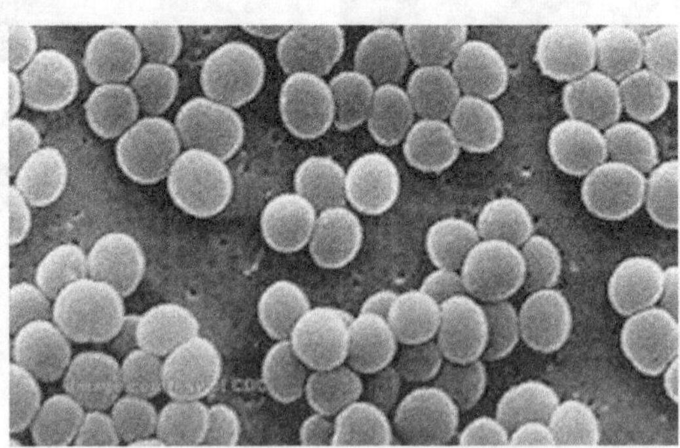

Structure of *Staphylococcus*

7. *Streptococcus*

Domain*: Bacteria*
Phylum*: Firmicutes*
Class*: Bacilli*
Order*: Lactobacillales*
Family*: Streptococcaceae*
Genus*: Streptococcus*

1. *Streptococci* are facultatively anaerobic, Gram positive, non-motile round shaped bacteria usually arranged in chains.

2. These bacteria are catalase test negative, in contrast *Staphylococci* are catalase positive.

3. *Streptococci* are of many groups and cause mild throat infections to pneumonia.

4. Few species form normal microbial flora of mouth, nose, intestine etc.

5. *Streptococci* are able to ferment sugars, but the end product is always lactic acid. Therefore, Streptococci are acid tolerant.

6. The presence of *Streptococci* in drinking water indicates fecal contamination.

7. Some of the examples of *Streptococcus* species are *S.pyogenes, S.bovis, S.mutans, S.pneumoniae etc.*

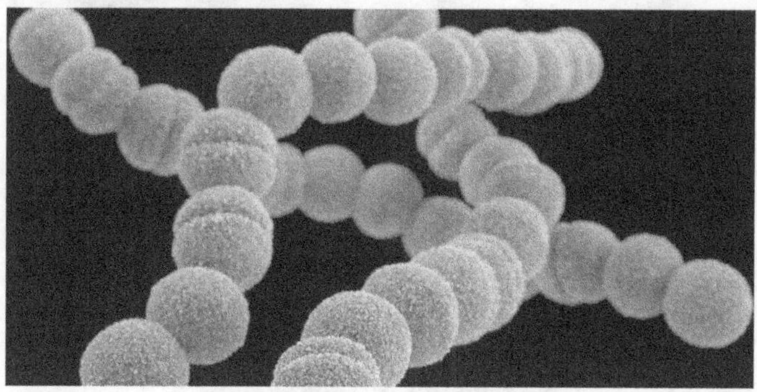

Structure of *Streptococcus*

8. *Salmonella*

> ***Domain****: Bacteria*
> ***Kingdom****: Eubacteria*
> ***Phylum****: Proteobacteria*
> ***Class****: Gammaproteobacteria*
> ***Order****: Enterobacteriales*
> ***Family****: Enterobacteriaceae*
> ***Genus****: Salmonella*

1. *Salmonella i*s a genus of Gram-negative, rod shaped, non-spore forming, motile, facutatively anaerobic bacteria.

2. They are oxidase, indole, Voges-Proskaur negative but catalase, methylred and Simmon citrate test positive.

3. *Salmonella* are found in intestine of human, warm and cold blooded animals and are shed through feces.

4. Humans become infected most frequently through contaminated water and food.

5. They are pathogenic to vertibrates and cause typhoid and enteric fever, septicaemia and gastroenteritis.

6. Some of the examples of species of *Salmonella* are *S.typhi*, *S.paratyphi*.

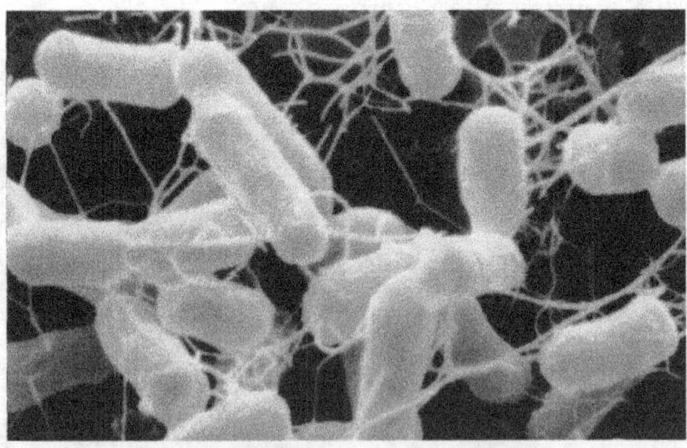

Structure of *Salmonella*

Suppliers of Microorganisms

Fungi

International Mycological Institute
Bakeham Lane, Egham, Surry TW 209, UK

American Type Culture Collection (ATCC)
P.O Box 1549
Manassas, VA 20108, USA

Carolina Biological Supply Company
Burlington, North Carolina 27215 USA

Centralbureau voor Schimmelcultures, CBS Fungal Biodiversity
Centre
P.O BOX-85167
NL-3508 AD Utrecht
Netherlands

BCCM/IHEM Culture Collection
Rue J, Wytsman straat 14
B-1050-Brussels,
Belgium

BCCM/ MUCL Culture Collection
    Croiok due sud 3
    B-1348
    Louvain-la-Neuve
    Belgium

    Microbial Type Culture Collection and Gene Bank (MTTC)
    CSIR-Institute of Microbial Technology
    Sector 39-A
    Chandigarh-160036, India

Yeasts

    BCCM/IHEM Culture Collection
    Rue J, Wytsman straat 14
    B-1050-Brussels,
    Belgium

Bacteria

    National Collection of Industrial bacteria (NCIB)
    Ferguson Building, Craibstone estate, Bucksburn
    Aberdeen AB 219YA, UK

    National Collection of Industrial Microorganisms (NCIM)
    National Chemical Laboratories
    Council of Scientific and Industrial Research (CSIR)
    Puna-8, India

Actinomycetes

    Scientific Research Institute of Search for New Antibiotics
    Russian Academy of Medical Sciences
    Bolshaia pirogovskaia 11, Moscow, Russia

9 789388 305020